SOTHIS PRESS

Sothis Press aims to completely reimagine the public domain book with an emphasis on universal access to captivatingly designed print editions. We believe that technology will enable every single book ever published to be perpetually accessible in beautiful print form. Sothis is beauty in ubiquity.

www.sothis.press
1 Waterhouse Square, London, ECIN 2ST

The Nervous Heart

Its Nature, Causation, Prognosis and Treatment

R. M. Wilson

SOTHIS PRESS

ISBN 978-1-0368-0773-3

This edition is published by
Sothis Press © 2023. The company
is registered in England and Wales.
The Company Number is 14900389.

THE NERVOUS HEART

ITS NATURE, CAUSATION, PROGNOSIS AND TREATMENT

BY

R. M. WILSON

CAPTAIN, R.A.M.C.

LATE ASSISTANT TO SIR JAMES MACKENZIE, UNDER THE MEDICAL RESEARCH COMMITTEE

CARDIOLOGIST TO THE TRENCH FEVER RESEARCH

AUTHOR OF "THE HEARTS OF MAN"

AND

JOHN H. CARROLL

MAJOR, M.C., U.S.A.

SPECIALLY ATTACHED TRENCH FEVER COMMITTEE

ASSISTANT VISITING PHYSICIAN, CITY HOSPITAL, NEW YORK

INSTRUCTOR, CLINICAL MEDICINE, UNIVERSITY AND BELLEVUE HOSPITAL MEDICAL COLLEGE

LONDON

HENRY FROWDE   HODDER & STOUGHTON

OXFORD UNIVERSITY PRESS   WARWICK SQUARE, E.C.

1919

PRINTED IN GREAT BRITAIN
BY MORRISON & GIBB LTD., EDINBURGH

PREFACE

THIS book is an attempt to view the problems of Heart Disease, and especially functional heart disease, from a new angle—that of the Nervous System.

There is no idea of opposing the views currently held regarding the efficiency of the myocardium and its bearing upon heart failure. But we venture to suggest that if a profound disturbance of the nervous control of the heart exists, the heart muscle will, on this account, work at a disadvantage. Its position will correspond to that of a motor engine when the controls and timing are out of order. The engine will not be able to develop its powers, and great strain will be put upon it.

With this explanation we offer our researches to the reader. We are very conscious of their many failings, and above all things we desire that we should not display a dogmatic spirit regarding them.

We desire to thank our Commanding Officer, Lieut.-Colonel T. S. Allan, for the help he has afforded us in showing every encouragement to scientific work, and we wish to express the great sense of indebtedness we feel to Major Wm. Byam, but for whose inspiration and enthusiasm this book would never have been written. We also record our thanks for much valuable criticism to Captain V. E. Sorapure.

R. M. WILSON.
JOHN H. CARROLL.

LONDON, *May* 1919.

CONTENTS

THE NERVOUS HEART

CHAPTER I

The Mechanism of the Emotions

The Reaction State and the Rest State.—In a previous work, *The Hearts of Man*, one of the present authors attempted to show that there are two sharp differentiations of physical function—the so-called reaction state, and the so-called rest state. The reaction state is the state of mental or muscular activity in which blood is driven from the great blood lakes or "hearts" (the peripheral lake, the pulmonary lake, and the mesenteric lake) and is forced at pressure into muscles and brain. In the reaction state all the hearts or lakes go into a condition of plus-systole, *i.e.*, the skin arterioles are vaso-constricted, the lung arterioles are vaso-constricted, the abdominal arterioles are vaso-constricted, the heart itself becomes smaller in size; the blood pressure in the great vessels rises; the muscles are engorged with blood, and the recti muscles are tense, acting by their thrust to drive blood out of both abdomen and thorax into the muscular field. The diaphragm is held in inhibition.

In the rest state, which follows reaction, invariably the exact opposite is seen. The hearts or lakes are open or in a condition of plus-diastole, the blood at easy pressure fills them, and the muscles are limp and flabby. The recti no longer carry on their thrust, and the diaphragm ascends and descends.

The Efficiency of Effort depends on the efficient emptying of the Blood Lakes.—Once the fact is grasped that the whole mechanism of reaction is a mechanism directed to filling the muscles with blood and the brain with blood, it becomes quite evident that the efficiency of any given effort, whether of the muscles or of the brain, depends upon the efficiency with which blood is driven into these structures. That efficiency depends primarily on the emptying of the great blood reservoirs—the skin, the belly, and the chest. If, for example, it be remembered that the mesenteric blood lake when fully dilated is capable of accommodating all the blood in the body it will be clear that should the mesenteric blood lake at any time remain fully dilated no blood could possibly be delivered to brain or muscles, and the patient would fall unconscious in a faint.

The Efficient Performance of Effort is therefore a Function of the Sympathetic Nervous System.—All the blood lakes are under nervous control. They are shut by the true or adrenalin sympathetic, and they are opened by the vagus depressor system. The same applies to the heart itself.

Consequently, during a call for effort, the true sympathetic dominates the picture, and the vagus depressor sympathetic is in a sense at least made subsidiary to it. The blood lakes are thus shut. If, however, from any cause the true sympathetic should be so weakened that it failed to produce active closing of the blood lakes, or, on the other hand, the vagus depressor system should be so strong that it at all times dominated the picture, the mechanism would break down. The blood lakes would not close and the muscles and brain would not be efficiently supplied. Clearly, then, any factor influencing the irritability of sympathetic nerves must influence also the efficiency of the reaction or effort state.

A **Hyper-Irritable Vagus Depressor System means Incomplete Effort.**—This evidently follows. If the vagus depressor system is in a state of hyper-excitability the blood lakes will not so easily be closed by the opposing true sympathetic mechanism. In popular language, it will "require an effort" to mobilize the blood needed for the muscles or brain, and during the whole period of the effort the exaggerated pull of the vagus depressor system will be felt. Thus an additional strain will be imposed on the true sympathetic mechanism, and when the effort ends there will be a tendency for a marked "swing back" into diastole to occur with, it may be, phenomena of fainting or collapse.

The Phenomenon of Fainting.—The phenomenon of fainting is easily understood if these considerations are borne in mind. It is essentially a vagus-depressor-system phenomenon. All the hearts or blood lakes open up together, so that the skin arterioles are dilated, the heart is dilated, the lung arterioles are dilated, and the mesenteric arterioles are dilated. At first the patient becomes uneasy, and may flush. Gradually, however, the immense mesenteric lake swallows up more and more blood. The blood flows out of the dilated skin lake, which becomes deadly pale, the pulse even disappears, the brain is emptied of blood and a *giddy sensation* results, the muscles are emptied of blood and a sense of *profound muscular weakness and exhaustion results.* The patient finally falls to the ground. Later, as the condition improves, the blood flows again into the open skin blood lake and a flush results. This is often spoken of as a vaso-dilatation. It is nothing of the sort. The vaso-dilatation of the skin was present from the outset. Only the blood was lacking to fill it.

The Pallor of Anger.—Very different from this picture is that of the pallor of anger, in which no sense of weakness or giddiness is experienced. On the contrary, the patient is ready to fight, and his muscles are strong and full of blood and his brain active. He is never pulseless.

In this case what we are viewing is a rapid and strong emptying of the skin lake owing to strong sympathetic action. This phenomenon is seen when an intravenous injection of adrenalin is given. The same thing is occurring in the other lakes, and so a large volume of blood is available for the muscles and brain.

The Emotions accompanying the Two Types of Pallor are very different.—If a careful study be made of the sensations and emotions accompanying the two types of pallor it will be found that whereas the man about to faint experiences fear, anxiety, and distress, the angry man experiences none of these feelings. Moreover, any improvement in his condition at once allays the anxiety of the fainting subject. His fear is proportional to his incapacity. Where complete capacity exists there is no fear.

It is therefore evident that with failure to mobilize the blood from the blood lakes is associated a sensation of fear, anxiety, depression, or distress, the extent of which depends on the extent of the failure.

When the mobilization of the blood is achieved, fear and depression pass away and are replaced, as in the case of the angry man, by confidence.

Fear, then, is a phenomenon of vagus depressor hyperexcitability; confidence is a phenomenon of true sympathetic activity.

The cases of the pallor of fainting and the pallor of anger are extreme cases. Between those extremes lie a vast number of examples of more or less distress and more or less confidence.

The Blush of Shame, or Nervousness.—This is a step on the way to fainting. The blood lakes are open, but not so greatly open that the blood can all be gathered in the mesenteric lake. Consequently a fine vaso-dilatation blush spreads over the skin. Patients who blush easily are usually of a "nervous" disposition.

When Vagus Dilator Phenomena show themselves in response to a Stimulus the Subject is always disturbed or confused in the First Instance.—This is a matter of observation. The blushing girl, the guilty boy, are obvious examples. So again is the employee face to face with an angry employer whom he dare not defy, the soldier face to face with his officer, and so on. In these instances the odds against action are too long, and inaction consequently prevails: the blood lakes are not emptied, the muscles are not filled.

In cases of disease where it can be shown that the vagus depressor mechanism is hyperexcitable through the action of some toxin, the same effect is produced when the odds against action are not normally long at all. The man is physically unable on account of his hyperexcitable vagus mechanism to mobilize his blood. He blushes and is disturbed and afraid.

In both cases, *i.e.* the case of the man who knows the odds are too long against action and the case of the man who is physically incapable of acting, the sense of disturbance which accompanies the event is more or less acute according as more or less failure to act takes place. Thus the greater the provocation the greater the distress, the greater the sense of weakness the greater the distress. And in both cases efforts will be made, *on a lower plane,* to relieve the distress in the only way in which it can be relieved, namely, by overcoming the vagus depressor mechanism and exercising the true sympathetic or reaction mechanism. The man who dared not face the long odds will be apt to ease his exasperation by angry demonstrations among his friends when his employer has gone away—he may "kick the dog." The sick man may—if he does not pass on to an actual faint—become excited and talkative, or laugh, or weep, or scold, or cough in a hysterical manner. But neither man will be able in this way to achieve complete satisfaction, and consequently both will remain irritable and exasperated. Irritation and exasperation are therefore also in an indirect way vagal depressor phenomena.

It will be readily understood that in other instances some sort of a reaction might be achieved. In the first instance, the employee might, for example, dare to speak plainly to his master; and the sick man might attempt to engage in hard effort. But the dice are weighted against both; in the one case by reason of external circumstances, in the other by reason of a toxæmia. Mobilization of blood is not effective; the vagus depressor system keeps its pull against the effort, and failure and irritation result.

The Meaning of Emotional Outbursts.—Emotional outbursts are therefore methods by which it is sought, on a lower plane, to overcome fear, distress, depression, or anxiety which have arisen because of the failure or partial failure of the true sympathetic system to dominate the vagus depressor system, whether from its own weakness, from weakness imposed upon it by circumstances, or from the exaggerated strength of the vagus mechanism, *e.g.* as the result of a toxæmia. These emotional outbursts may take the form of rage, or irritability, of laughing or crying or coughing fits, of yawning, or of hysterical attacks of a more active kind. In all these cases the picture of reaction is imitated: the glottis is closed, or closed and opened in jerks, the abdominal muscles contract, and blood is thrust out of the lakes into the muscular field and brain. A sense of relief is afforded. This aspect of the question has been carefully studied and elucidated by Crile, to whose work the authors express their indebtedness.

The Picture of Incapacity.—The picture of incapacity is therefore the picture of vagus depressor activity with the picture of reaction superimposed on it to a greater or a less degree, but always to a lesser degree than the circumstances of the moment demand—that is to say, the picture of exhaustion. It is characterized by giddiness, weakness, breathlessness, pain, especially over the heart, a weak form of excitement, tremulousness, sweating, blushing, and palpitation. The effort has been made and has not sufficed. Subsidiary efforts are going on, *e.g.* crying—to attempt on a lower plane what was not achieved on a higher.

CHAPTER II

The Principle of Compensation

THE law just enunciated, that if failure to react fully upon a high plane occurs, reaction on a lower plane will be attempted, is a law of life, as a little consideration will show. No less fully is it a law of life that failure to react to the full extent with its accompanying emotions, fear, anxiety, grief, or sorrow, inflicts upon the organism such distress that either some means must be found to remove the memory or the circumstances of the failure, or else a mechanism of compensation must be called in to overcome the inability and enable reaction to take place.

The Meaning of Forgetfulness.—It is not proposed to go deeply into the mental processes involved, but it is clear that in forgetfulness a mechanism exists whereby the memory of failure to react fully and normally can be lost or buried. In its extreme forms forgetfulness may amount to a total loss of individuality, *e.g.* in shell shock, to loss of sensation, to loss of one of the special senses, and so on. In these cases the individual admits failure, renounces for the time the possibility in this instance of compensating his weakness by strength, and, so far as he can, "cuts his loss." Modern psychological medicine is built up on the recognition of this fact. What is often lost sight of is that many so-called neurotic or hysterical people are the victims of a toxæmia which renders their vagus depressor mechanism unduly active and so prevents them from reacting normally. They are physically unfit for courageous actions, because they cannot in circumstances of great stress close their blood lakes and so cannot obtain the needful blood supply to their muscles. Every time an effort is demanded, failure occurs with fear and distress, until at last they perceive that only in forgetfulness of their "cowardice" can relief be found. These patients therefore seek reaction on a lower plane, often by convincing themselves that they suffer from diseases (which in point of fact they do), by worrying about these diseases, by worrying about their circumstances, their friends—anything, everything. It is all that is left to them to do, and they are as really ill in a purely physical or organic sense as a man with pneumonia.

Compensation and Training.—In everyday life man constantly puts into practice the law of compensation, in order that he may "rise superior to circumstances" and achieve the—for him—hitherto impossible. The drill sergeant who turns recruits into good fighting material is an exponent of this law, and his methods are worth watching because they afford a demonstration of the mechanism of the reaction state.

On parade a soldier is instructed to hold himself erect, to throw back his shoulders, stick out his chest, and draw in his abdomen. In other words, he is instructed to empty his abdominal blood lake, to make his chest funnel-shaped so that the thrust of his recti muscles may drive the blood out of it as well as out of his abdomen, and to put his muscles in the best position for effort when they are filled with blood, as they must be in these circumstances.

The result of this training is an increase of "tone"—in other words, an increase in the ability of the blood lakes or hearts to contract rapidly and at given words of command, and so an increase in reaction efficiency. Effort becomes "easier," more automatic, less laborious. The confusion and mental disturbance attending the early stages of training are overcome, confidence is acquired, and fear and anxiety got rid of.

Every one is familiar with this picture, so much so that the statement "courage is a matter of habit" has been made. More true it would be to say that any act accomplished without distress is an act during the performance of which the vagus depressor mechanism is fully compensated by the sympathetic mechanism. The adequate compensation of the vagus depressor by the sympathetic is the victory over circumstances spoken of by lay writers. The same man, evidently, may perform one act without distress, and yet suffer great distress in another act in the performance of which his sympathetic mechanism proves unequal to a vagus depressor stimulated to an unwonted degree by special circumstances, *e.g.* memory pictures, a sense of guilt, disinclination, and so on, even though this second act is of a less strenuous character. This applies equally to sick men. The writer has seen cases in which a sick man suffered acute distress on slight effort to which he was unaccustomed or which he did not desire to carry out (route-marching in soldiers) yet could easily perform heavier work which he wished to carry out. His whole plane of response was lower owing to a hyperexcitable vagus depressor system, but the variations seen in the normal were seen also in him. These variations are well known to every one, and the expression "Where there's a will there's a way" puts the matter in concise language so far as everyday life is concerned.

Compensation in Disease.—Disease, in the sense in which it is understood by the public, means a failure to accomplish life without distress. It is this very failure which brings the patient to the doctor, and what the patient is concerned about is not what his exact illness may be, but whether or not he can get free from his distress and so be able to resume his normal functional efficiency.

In a number of instances the patient comes to the doctor with symptoms comparable to those of the man who, in good health, fails to react or who is prevented from complete reaction by the hyperexcitability of his vagus depressor mechanism.

This observation led the authors to investigate a number of disease conditions with a view to detecting the hyperirritability or otherwise of the vagus depressor mechanism. The work was begun on so-called "trench fever" because they happened to be engaged on the study of that disease at the time, but they have since observed very similar phenomena to those about to be described in septic infections, tonsillitis, diphtheria, splenomedullary leukæmia, rheumatic conditions, rheumatoid arthritis (Figs. 1 and 2).

Testing the Irritableness of the Vagus Depressor Mechanism.—It was accidentally found that if a long breath be taken and held, marked slowing of the pulse or a marked fall in pulse volume results in certain subjects. In other subjects no such slowing occurs, or a quickening may occur.

A number of normal controls (all cases with a history of rheumatic fever, "rheumatism," or any recent infection of any kind being excluded) were at once obtained, eight in number, and of these only one showed any slowing or any fall in volume, and that only to the extent of five

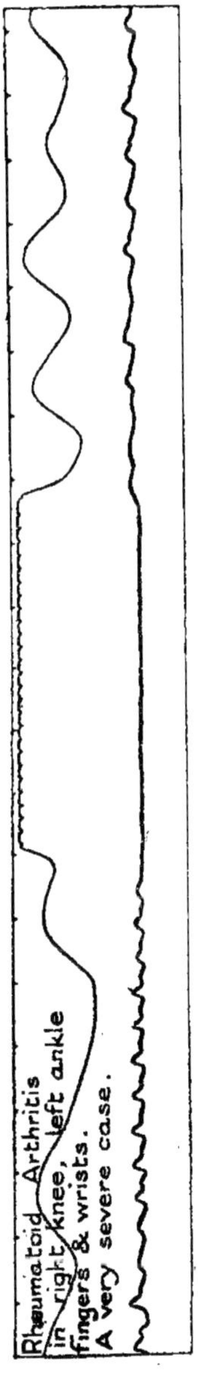

FIG. 1.—Note disappearance of pulse on deep inspiration.

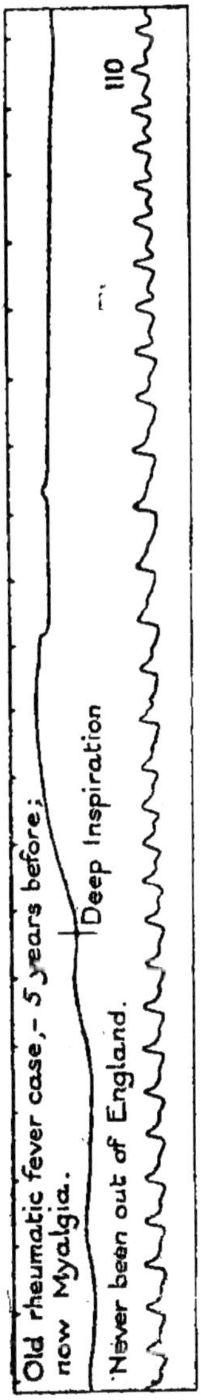

FIG. 2.—Note the marked slowing and augmented beating on deep inspiration.

beats per minute. The patients showing the slowing often slowed to thirty and even forty beats per minute (Figs. 3, 4, and 5).

The next step was to examine a number of

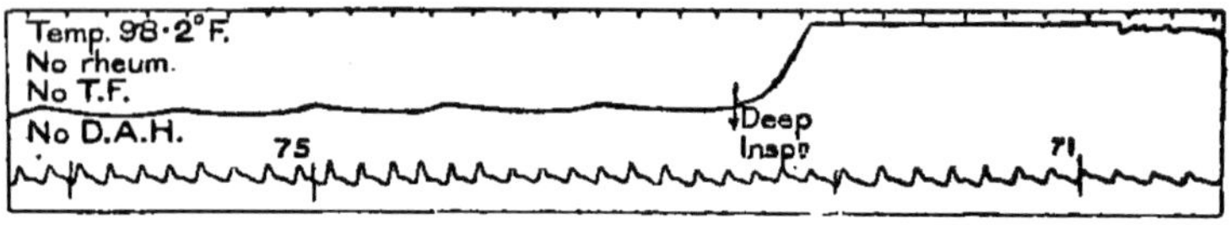

FIG. 3.—Normal Control. No slowing, no loss of volume on deep inspiration.

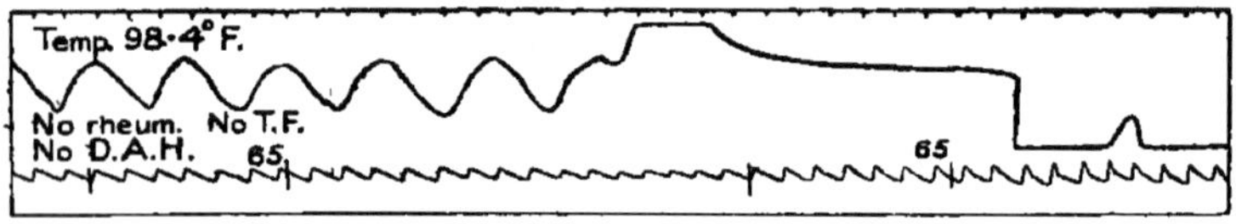

FIG. 4.—Another Normal Control. No slowing and no loss of volume on deep inspiration.

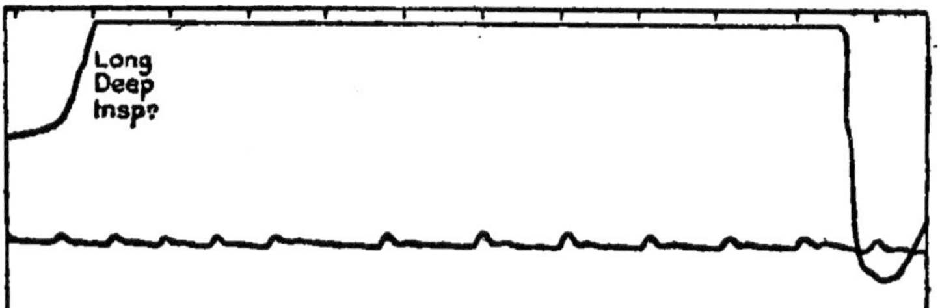

FIG. 5.—Trench Fever. Marked slowing on deep inspiration.

apparently healthy boys. Sixty-one of these were tested in this way, and it was found that of the 61, 42 showed no slowing of the pulse nor any loss of volume, while 19 showed slowing or loss of volume. Of the 42 not one had suffered from any previous illness. The histories of the 19 are as follows (all the boys were eighteen years old):—

1. Scarlet fever in childhood and typhoid fever four years ago.
2. Acne all over back and shoulders. No history of disease.
3. Diphtheria ten years ago.
4. Slight acne of back. Markedly nervous during examination. No history of disease.
5. (Slight slowing.) Scarlet fever. The hands of this patient were very blue.
6. Scarlet fever at ten years.
7. Tubercular glands removed. Scars present.
8. Scarlet fever in early life.
9. No history. (Slight slowing.)
10. No history. (Slight slowing.)
11. Tonsillitis at examination.
12. Deformed chest, old rachitis.
13. (Slight slowing.) Series of nasal operations on turbinate bones.
14. Pulse rate 160 at examination. Swollen glands in neck, the nature of which was not determined.
15. "Rheumatic" subject.
16. (Slight case.) Severe attack some years ago of synovitis in knee.
17. Curious hard scaly skin which he said

was hereditary. (This condition amounted to a gross deformity.)

18. Scarlet fever some years ago. Some extra systoles noted.

19. Scarlet fever. Systolic murmur present.

These results fully confirmed other results obtained at other periods. The conclusion was that in quite healthy persons with clear histories slowing was not usually met with; when it was encountered the history contained a record of some illness. Further, the functional efficiency of these boys was less than normal. They admitted in a majority of cases to some dyspnœa on exertion. Finally it was found in a series of hospital cases that $\frac{1}{33}$ grain of atropine given subcutaneously always removed the slowing and loss of volume (see below) (Figs. 6, 7, and 8), thus indicating that the phenomenon was vagal and depressor in origin.

But not only Slowing was encountered, Loss of Pulse Volume was also encountered.—In the cases tested, loss of pulse volume was at least as common as slowing (Figs. 6 and 7). It tended to appear if the breath taken was especially deep or if it was held a long time. Sometimes it was so great that the pulse disappeared completely (so-called "pulsus paradoxus"), at other times it was less complete. Sometimes the slowing preceded it, sometimes followed it. It was likewise abolished or lessened by atropine.

The phenomenon is evidently, as has been said,

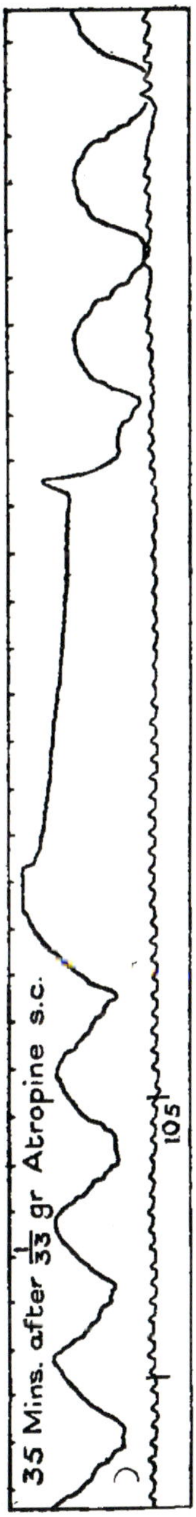

FIG. 6.—Effect of Atropine on Pulse, which disappeared on deep inspiration.

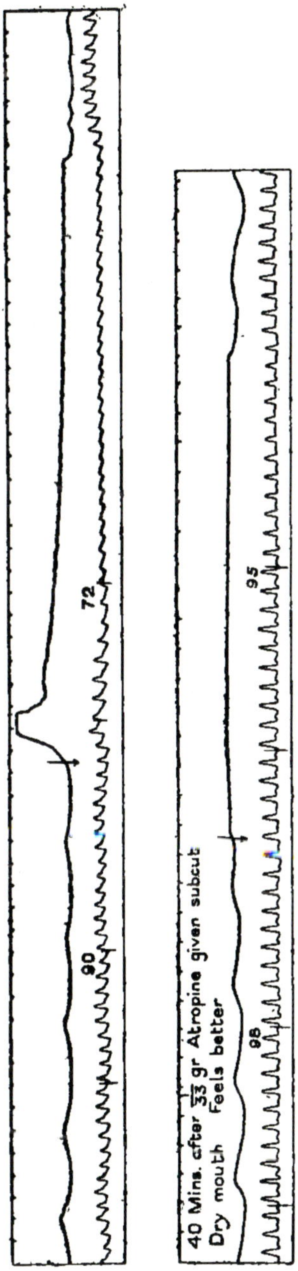

FIG. 7.—Effect of Atropine on Pulse, the volume of which fell sharply on deep inspiration.

a vagus depressor one; it is quite evident that it is caused by so great an opening of the abdominal

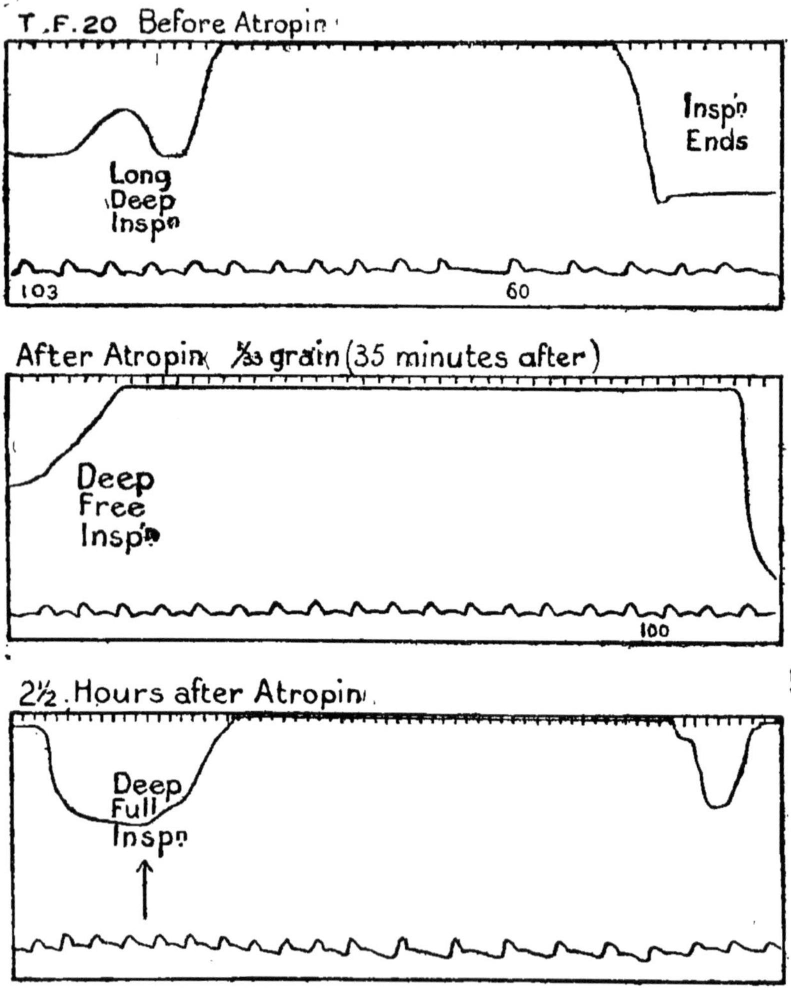

FIG. 8.—Slowing of Pulse on Deep Inspiration, removed by Atropine.

and pulmonary blood lakes under stimulation of the vagus depressor system, that the blood volume in the periphery is lowered or cut down to nothing.

When the Vagus Depressor Mechanism is overactive, a Compensatory Mechanism is brought into play.—This must necessarily occur, or life and activity could not be maintained. If an overacting vagus be present then the sympathetic system must likewise overact, or the patient will be unable to perform the actions of life. In the genesis of so-called "functional heart disease" this mechanism is seen at work, as we shall hope to show in the succeeding chapters.

CHAPTER III

The Genesis of Functional Heart Disease

ONE of the authors spent about two years studying the condition known as the Irritable Heart of Soldiers or Disordered Action of the Heart (D.A.H.), first as Cardiologist, under Sir James Mackenzie, at Fulham Military Hospital and later at the Hampstead Military Hospital for the Study of Diseases of the Heart in Soldiers, of the Research Department of which Dr. Thomas Lewis was head. The cardinal symptoms of this condition were very clearly marked, but proved difficult of analysis and explanation. They were : breathlessness on exertion, palpitation, pain over the præcordium, and giddiness. These symptoms tended to come on when effort was attempted and they disappeared as a rule when the patient lay at ease in bed. They were thus effort symptoms, and for this reason Dr. Lewis named the condition the *effort syndrome.*

Patients with Irritable Heart are Patients in a Chronic State of Exhaustion.—During the course of the study of irritable heart Sir James Mackenzie expressed the view to one of the authors that the symptoms of the patients with irritable heart were the symptoms of exhaustion met with in any man who has overexerted himself or otherwise drawn too far on his natural resources.

The more closely the soldiers were studied the more evident did it become that this view was correct. The men were incapable of effort evidently because they lived in the kind of state which normally is produced by too much effort. They sweated excessively; they became breathless on slight provocation, they trembled, they felt giddy and irritable and "rotten." They seemed to be unable to stand long on their feet. They often fainted. All of them complained of a sense of great weakness and exhaustion. Some had enlarged thyroids, many presented features associated in the professional mind with hyperthyroidism.

Both True Sympathetic and Vagus Depressor Sympathetic are hyperexcitable in Patients with Irritable Heart.—In company with Captain Francis R. Fraser one of the authors administered to a series of these patients and to a series of healthy controls a dose of adrenalin intravenously. The patients reacted much more violently to the drug than did the controls. *The conclusion was drawn that the true sympathetic system was hyperexcitable in those patients.*

Next, apocodeine, which Dixon has shown to be a drug exercising an inhibitory effect on the true sympathetic, was administered to patients and controls. The patients reacted violently: the controls did not react. *The conclusion was drawn that the vagus system was hyperexcitable in these patients* (several of the patients flushed all over the skin in a most remarkable way). *At first it appeared to be very difficult to see why both systems should be hyperexcitable in these cases.*[1]

The Causal Agent in Irritable Heart.—Meanwhile attempts to find the causal agent of irritable heart had been made and had failed. One thing, however, had emerged. " Irritable heart " was not one separate entity: it marked the convalescent stage of many acute conditions, *e.g.* dysentery, pneumonia, septic poisonings, and in certain instances it passed off completely. In other instances it did not pass off. Colonel Meakins, one of the workers at the Heart Hospital, was able to show that cases of irritable heart following amœbic dysentery, the stools of which were reported free from *Entamœba histolytica* as the result of treatment by bismuth-emetine-iodide, tended to recover from their irritable hearts.

At this point Major Byam, the officer in charge of the Medical Division at the hospital, invited one of the authors to study trench fever cases side by side with the cases of irritable heart.

Trench Fever as a Cause of Irritable Heart.—The upshot of this study was the conviction that some 80 per cent. at least of all cases of irritable heart

[1] *B.M.J.*, July 1918.

in soldiers are due to the infection of trench fever, the remaining percentages being distributed among diseases of which "rheumatism" and dysentery are probably the most important.

The Nervous Phenomena in Trench Fever.—The onset of trench fever is usually marked by great muscular weakness and often by collapse and fainting. It was soon determined that in early cases of the disease the vagus depressor system was greatly overexcited. Marked slowing of the pulse occurred on deep inspiration in some cases; in others rapidity with marked loss of pulse volume, frequently true pulsus paradoxus or total disappearance of the radial pulse. These phenomena could always be removed by atropine with conspicuous, though very temporary, relief to the patient.

The Symptoms of Hyperthyroidism.—Reference has already been made to the view that hyperthyroidism plays a part in the picture of functional heart disease. This view has found many supporters, both before and since the outbreak of war. It is evidently founded upon the fact that patients suffering from this condition show, as a rule, profuse sweating, flushing, and tremulousness.

The theory was strongly advanced in 1915 especially, and was urged by, among others, Sir James Barr of Liverpool and Dr. Florence Stoney of the Fulham Military Hospital. It was disputed, notably by Lewis, who found that the administration of thyroid extract by no means tended to exaggerate the symptoms ascribed to thyroid overactivity, a state of matters which, he suggested, might have been expected had hyperthyroidism been the basis of the syndrome.

The authors extended Lewis's work, and found in addition that, far from exaggerating the symptoms, large doses of thyroid extract distinctly and definitely cause relief. This finding has been confirmed on so many cases and with such uniformity that the beneficial effects of thyroid are certainly not an accident. The following are instances of what is meant :—

Case 1.—On the forty-sixth day of disease (trench fever) patient developed marked sensations of exhaustion, shakiness, profuse sweating, and dyspnœa on exertion. The pulse was rapid.

Patient was put on thyroid 2 grains thrice daily, and immediately thereafter the symptoms disappeared.

A week later the thyroid was discontinued and the symptoms returned, with a tendency to fainting, severe headache, and giddiness. A further course of thyroid was begun, and all symptoms again disappeared. On again being taken off thyroid, the symptoms returned.

Case 2.—On the thirtieth day of disease (trench fever) patient developed profuse sweating, marked tremor, dizziness, headache, and tachycardia. He was then put on thyroid 2 grains three times a day, and at once got rid of his symptoms. Treatment in this case was not discontinued, and the patient remains well.

This experience was met with even in cases which showed definite thyroid enlargement, as the following clearly demonstrates :—

Case 3.—In this case thyroid enlargement and discomfort in the neck accompanied the appearance of irritable heart symptoms. This patient could take 9 grains of thyroid daily without ill effect, indeed with comfort, for he improved steadily while taking it.

The Onset of Irritable Heart is usually seen about Three Weeks or a Month after the beginning of the Acute Illness.—It must not be understood that the results of the use of thyroid in cases of irritable heart following trench fever have led to the conclusion formulated by Lewis, namely, that the thyroid gland plays no part in the mechanism of this condition. The most striking feature of the majority of early cases of trench fever is the disinclination of the patient to respond to calls for effort. This disinclination is no local weakness of the legs, but a general extreme exhaustion accompanied by fainting in many cases and by bradycardia. At this point, as has been suggested, the vagus depressor mechanism is in a high state of excitability, and the patient is literally without the power to relieve himself of the depressing effect produced—*i.e.* he cannot close his blood lakes and so cannot obtain the muscular blood supply requisite for much effort.

A fallacy is apt to creep in here and to upset the clear view of the condition that is essential. The fallacy is this. After the first acute attack with fever has passed away, the patient, while lying in bed, suffers as a rule no marked distress. He attempts nothing except trivial movements, and these he performs easily. It is when he gets up that distress, dyspnœa, etc., begins—*that is to say, when effort is attempted.*

If, however, his first attack be studied it will be observed that he suffered distress at the beginning, marked distress, *while he still attempted to carry on his work in spite of his condition.* At that time he was breathless and giddy and had pains over his heart, just as he has later on rising from bed to resume his life. In fact, in many instances complete collapse took place before he went to hospital in the first instance.

Again, if the attack was a severe one, he suffered still another attack of distress in his bed in hospital, when he "felt too weak even to sit up in the bed." That distress caused him to be breathless while lying in bed, and the breathlessness was apt to occur during the night. The moment we remember that even the simplest activities of life *depend for their successful accomplishment on an adequate sympathetic response to vagus depressor "pull,"* we see that for any given effort, no matter how small, there is a minimal degree of sympathetic activity. If the vagus depressor system is so irritable as the result of toxic action that it cannot in a given case be adequately responded to, the particular effort attempted will be impossible. Smaller efforts may still be possible in these circumstances, but not without great expenditure of sympathetic activity—that is to say, without great "strain." The patient in these cases may be rendered breathless by turning in bed, and he may even be breathless without moving, because of the "effort" required to live at all and keep up such a tonic state of his blood lakes as will enable his brain to receive the minimum nourishment necessary for its life. A good illustration of this is seen in the later stages of severe illness when the patient performs reaction breathing not in order to do work, but in order to live.

Consequently a law emerges: *Symptoms of distress and dyspnœa appear every time that the means to accomplish any end fall short of the necessity of the case, whether the end be merely lying at rest in bed, moving about in bed, or performing strenuous exercise.*

As the patient "recovers," his life in bed becomes easy, because he has now no difficulty in finding the power for all the efforts required of him. But when he gets up for the first time he is once more face to face with distress and difficulty—the assumption of the erect posture is in itself enough to cause collapse in some cases.

The Capacity of the Patient now depends on the Extent of the Irritability of his Vagus Depressor System, on the power of response of his Sympathetic System, and on a Host of External Conditions which we may call collectively "Circumstances" (an example of these latter was, during the war, the desire of many men to avoid returning to the firing line).—Not one of these three factors can be separated from the others, and most of the mistakes made in regard to functional heart conditions have arisen because an attempt to separate them has been made. Thus, if the condition of the vagus depressor mechanism alone be considered, the cases are apt to be treated from a neurological point of view, or even from a purely cardiological point of view. The neurologist is, however, always painfully aware that there are signs and symptoms which lie outside the strict picture, and he is not able to refute the claims of the cardiologist on the one hand or the psychotherapist on the other. Nor can the cardiologist refute his claims.

On the other hand, attempts to regard the condition as due to "sympathetic exhaustion" end as a rule in disaster, because it is easy to show that in many of these cases the sympathetic system is not exhausted—for example, the man who appears ready to collapse on the drill ground may often be seen later *running* without distress, or walking out cheerfully with his sweetheart. It is just here, as we have attempted to show earlier, that external circumstances have their bearing on the problem as they have their bearing on all human problems. Nevertheless, those who seek the complete explanation in the mental field are likely to miss a true understanding.

These difficulties, we insist, disappear if the law we have enunciated is borne always in mind, namely: **Symptoms of distress and dyspnœa appear every time that the means to accomplish any end fall short of the necessity** of **the case, whether the end be merely lying at rest in bed, moving about in bed,** or **performing strenuous exercise.**

This, it will be seen, covers all cases—the cases in which an external cause, such as military discipline, weighs the dice in favour of the vagus depressor "pull" and against the sympathetic response to that "pull," and so prevents mobilization in an adequate manner of blood to muscles and brain; the cases in which an exhausted sympathetic system fails to respond adequately to the calls of a normal vagus, *e.g.* the tired man; and finally, the cases in which an hyperexcited vagus upon which a toxin is acting prevents the adequate response of the sympathetic, *e.g.* trench fever, "rheumatism," and so on.

It will further be seen that under this law symptoms of so-called irritable heart may occur in the case of any man several times a day, each time in fact that his activities or circumstances prevent him from making an adequate response to stimuli whether in the shape of provocations or calls for commonplace efforts. The picture of fear, mortification, or chagrin is not only like the picture of functional heart disease, it is the same picture; the differences that occur are differences in degree. That is to say, the victim of functional heart disease has a more irritable vagus than the normal man to start with. He is subject in every other respect to the same conditions. The soldier who fears the task ahead of him and who is called "nervous" is suffering in a lesser degree from a group of symptoms which, when he has contracted trench fever and been classed as a D.A.H. case, he will suffer from more acutely. The thought of danger in his toxic state will continue to exercise its effect upon him just as it did before he became toxic, but because his vagus depressor mechanism is now more active, the effect will now be more pronounced.

Distress occurs only when Effort is attempted—that is to say, only when the Sympathetic Mechanism is called upon to respond to the Vagus Depressor Mechanism.—This follows from the above. So long as a man attempts no effort above his powers,—that is, attempts no effort in which his sympathetic is not able to respond adequately to his vagus depressor mechanism and so achieve the needful blood supply to the brain and muscles,—just so long is he free from distress. The moment the sympathetic fails of adequate response, no matter from what cause, symptoms of distress appear. It will be readily understood that an increase in the excitability of the vagus depressor mechanism must therefore tend to "limit the field of response" by raising the degree of response which the sympathetic mechanism must afford.

The Vagus Depressor Mechanism sets the Pace of Response to Stimuli or of Reaction.—Life is an expression of the interrelation of pressor and depressor activities, of sympathetic and vagus depressor activities. Life is impossible in circumstances in which one or other of these mechanisms is put out of commission for any length of time. The writers recently witnessed an accident at a baseball match in which the "striker" was hit over the abdomen by the ball. He fell in a heap, evidently either as the result of a momentary paralysis of the sympathetic mechanism controlling and closing the abdominal blood lake or of a stimulation of the vagus depressor mechanism—in other words, he was "hit in the wind" and suffered such "loss of breath" that he could not stand. The vagus depressor mechanism had him in full grip.

In every function of life, then, the two mechanisms are at work, in relation to one another, and normally the response required of the sympathetic would seem to be determined by the vagus.

The mechanism of this vagus depressor governing action is not clear unless it be borne in mind that the abdominal blood lake, like the heart, goes into systole and diastole (see, for proofs, *The Hearts of Man*). By increasing diastole, therefore, a greater succeeding systole is determined. Gradually in succeeding beats systole predominates over diastole, that is to say, relaxation becomes smaller and smaller at each succeeding beat, and the whole blood lake passes into a condition of *plus-systole.*

The work of Roget[1] deserves to be quoted here, it being borne in mind that the sympathetic nervous system—as opposed to the vagus depressor system—is activated by adrenalin :—

" When, in a normal rabbit, we excite, by a faradic current, the peripheral end of the cut vagus, we observe a true stoppage of the heart, that is to say, a diastolic fall, sharp and profound, which is almost always followed by a return of the beats. The curve resulting is V-shaped. The first excitation always produces the most marked effect.

" If now we carry out the experiment on a decapsulated rabbit the first tracing obtained looks like a normal tracing, but during the second faradization the stoppage of the heart is prolonged and the return of the beat is made with difficulty.

" Continuing our excitations we soon obtain diastolic periods lasting as long as 30 or even 40 seconds. . . .

" How are we to explain these differences ? We might say generally that the vagus in the

[1] Roget, *Presse Medicale,* Nov. 22, 1917, " Quelques Recherches Recentes sur les Functions des Capsules Surrenales."

normal rabbit shows less and less effect in repeated stimulations because it is becoming exhausted. If this was the correct explanation we should find the same phenomenon in the decapsulated rabbit. But since in the decapsulated rabbit exactly the reverse is found, we are forced to take into consideration the only element that differs in the two series of experiments—the suprarenal capsules. We thus arrive at the following conception :—

"When the action of the vagus becomes preponderant, when it acts, that is to say, with full force on the heart, a reaction probably of the

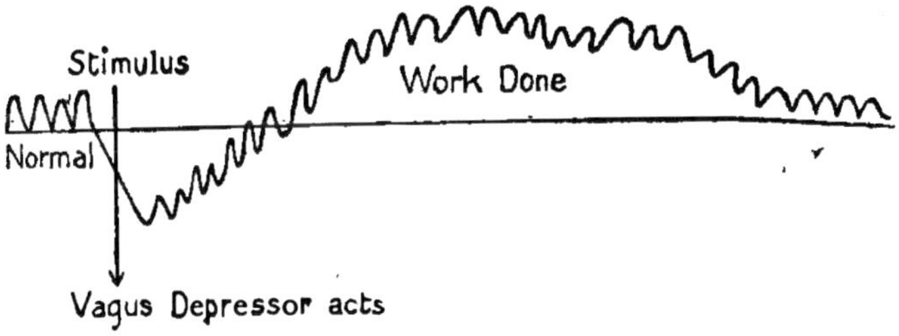

FIG. 9.—Illustrating the Normal Pressor Response to a Stimulus.

nature of a reflex is produced on the suprarenal capsules, which give out adrenalin. This adrenalin counterbalances the action of the vagus, prevents the stoppage of the heart, and raises the arterial pressure."

Roget, it will be seen, has arrived at the same view as the writers so far as the heart itself is concerned. This passage of the abdominal and other "hearts" into plus-systole as a response of a compensatory kind to vagus pull which was fully discussed in *The Hearts of Man*, is the key to the problem we are studying. In Fig. 9 we see this diagrammatically. A stimulus occurs. The vagus pulls. Pressure falls. Reaction at once occurs, the sympathetic responding; strong systoles follow the strong diastoles of the pulling vagus. Gradually the sympathetic mechanism swings the pendulum over and the abscissa rises. The lakes or hearts pass into plus-systole, arterial pressure rises above normal, the muscles and brain receive their increased supply of blood, and the effort necessitated by the given stimulus is accomplished.

If, however, the vagus pull happens for any reason to be greatly exaggerated, then it will follow either that—

(1) The patient will collapse without making any response, and no effort will be accomplished at all, or

(2) The response will be inadequate to the pull—the subsequent rise will not suffice to the effort required or may even fail to reach the original abscissa so that the latter state of the man is worse than the first (Figs. 10 and 11).

In these cases distress will accompany the failure to respond in an adequate manner, and response on a lower plane may be attempted in order to "ease exasperation," or, in other words, put an end to the distressful clash of mechanisms which should be working harmoniously.

We may thus say that reaction to a given stimulus will vary according to the state of the vagus depressor mechanism. If this mechanism is very excessively excitable, the patient may faint and may not react. If the mechanism is rather less excitable, the patient may "feel faint" and may react so little that, as he says himself in these

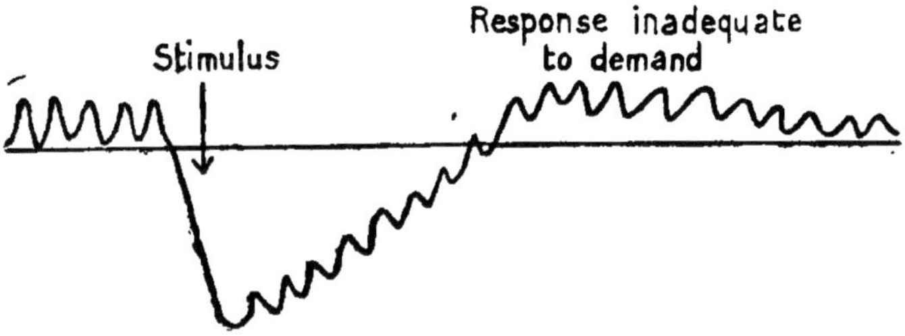

FIG. 10.—Illustrating the Pressor Response to a Stimulus when the Vagus is overactive.

cases, "When I try to do anything I am done for" (Fig. 12). If the mechanism is still rather less excitable, the patient may merely fail to

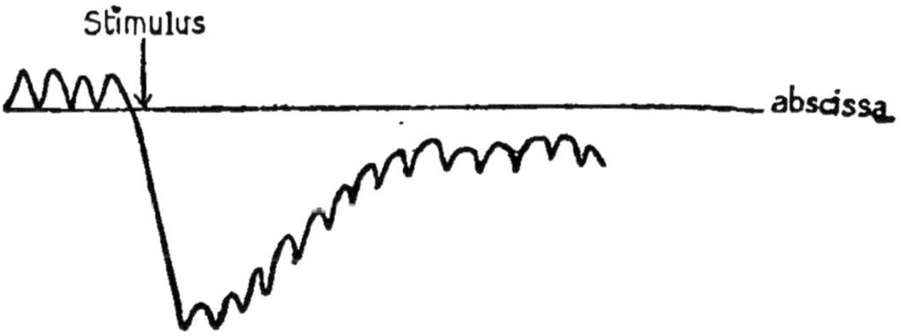

FIG. 11.—A More Advanced Stage of Vagus Overexcitability.

achieve the necessary degree of reaction, and recognizing this failure may react on a lower level—what we have called "kicking the dog." Finally, if the vagus is normal and the stimulus not excessive, reaction of a normal kind will occur. Necessarily the more irritable the vagus the more every small stimulus will affect it, and consequently the more excessive the demand for reaction will be. This will rapidly tire the patient out and exhaust his resources, thus speedily in another direction restricting his "field of response." It must never for an instant, on the other hand, be forgotten that reaction varies also with the stimulus, and that stimuli are no simple phenomena, but are

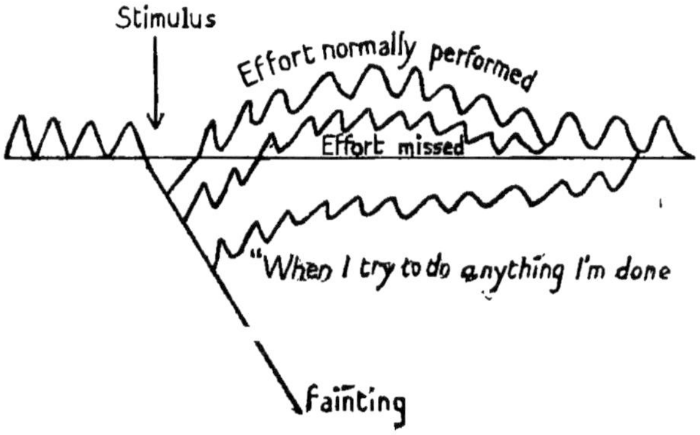

FIG. 12.—Illustrating the Pressor Responses in Various Stages of Vagus Hyperexcitability.

almost invariably made up of complex personal associations. The sound of a gun may mean nothing to one man; in the case of another man it may conjure up terrible mental images, which reinforce the effect of the stimulus a thousandfold and so produce a vagus depressor pull out of all proportion.

The Determining Factor of Vagus Depressor Activity is well understood by the Ordinary Man.—The layman who speaks from his own experience pays constant and valuable tribute to the part played by the vagus depressor mechanism in determining reaction. "My heart stood still" is a common description of the effect of a sudden shock or stimulus. "Took my breath away" is another. "My heart sank," another (a good description of the sudden opening of the abdominal blood lake).

"I turned hot and cold" is a good description of general vaso-dilatation followed by a gradual concentration of blood in the abdominal lake, and so its disappearance from the periphery; "You could have knocked me down with a feather" expresses the muscular weakness which occurs.

In the Normal Man the Response to Vagal Action is instant and powerful, so that Reaction appears to be continuous with Normal Life.—The healthy man lives in a state of preparation for reaction, and possesses abundant and easily realized power to react. His vagus depressor mechanism not being unduly excited does not in ordinary circumstances impose an undue response upon his sympathetic system.

Moreover, the oftener the same stimulus occurs the more rapid and perfect will be the response to it in ordinary healthy people. That is to say, the determining vagus "pull" regarding it will get less, the amount of response will be more exactly adjusted to the need of the situation—by this time a familiar one—and the reaction will be carried out with the minimum of effort. The task of yesterday will have become the easy accomplishment of to-day. This is the underlying principle of habit, of getting accustomed to things, of spending the minimum of effort to achieve a given purpose.

It is evident that to increase the excitability of the vagus by a toxin is to upset this delicate adjustment of means to end, to demand a greater degree of reaction for every task, no matter how familiar, to put a tax on all resources. The victim of vagus hyperexcitability will of course still be able to accomplish his own special task more easily than any other task, but even his own special task will now demand greater expenditures of energy than in the days of health.

An Increase in the Irritability of the Vagus Depressor Mechanism imposes a Reconstruction of Nervous Balance.—It is obvious that any increase of vagus excitability will entail, if life is to be lived on the same plane as before, a corresponding increase of sympathetic excitability. Only when this has been achieved will the organism be able to accomplish the necessary reactions of everyday life without distress and trouble.

In the trench fever cases it was found that after a time, even though the vagus system of the patients was not less excitable than it had been at the onset of the disease, the response to effort underwent improvement—in other words, the patient was able, by means of some mechanism he had brought into play, to compensate for the hyperexcitability of his vagus mechanism when an effort was required of him.

A lead in the direction of the nature of this compensation was afforded by the fact that in some cases enlargement of the thyroid gland was met with and phenomena usually associated with hyperthyroidism encountered.

These phenomena, coupled with the good effects of thyroid administration, suggested the conclusion that the so-called "hyperthyroidism" met with in these cases is in the nature of a compensation to the depressor effects of vagus hyperexcitability.

The work of Canon, Cattell, and Levy has demonstrated that the mechanism of pressor effects, as opposed to depressor, involves the suprarenals and the thyroid. Canon and Cattell place the secretory innervation of the thyroid on a firm basis in a work appearing in July 1916 (*Amer. Journal of Physiology*). They show that thyroid secretion resulted from stimulation of the cervical sympathetic nerve and also from adrenal injection, the latter through the blood stream. That is to say, that at times of sympathetic and of adrenal activity a call will be made upon the thyroid secretion.

It is well recognized that vagal stimulation with its resulting depression calls for adrenal or sympathetic activity (see the work of Roget, quoted above). Consequently the normal reaction of a man to excessive excitability of his vagus system will be a mobilization of adrenalin and thyroid, and so a reaction based upon the sympathetic system.

Adrenalin, as is well known, acts by constricting splanchnic arterioles and so closing the dilated splanchnic lake. A marked pressor effect results. Indeed, Hoskins has shown that the pressor effect of adrenalin depends entirely upon the emptying of this blood lake, since, if the splanchnic area be excluded from the circulation, adrenalin no longer is able to produce any pressor effect. Levy has conclusively proved that the pressor effect of adrenalin is multiplied from 200 to 300 per cent. if thyroid be present.

It therefore follows that if the blood stream contains an excess of thyroid less adrenalin will be required for any given pressor effect, or, in other words, the accelerator and other effects of adrenalin will be less evident in these cases, and effort will be accompanied by a smaller degree of tachycardia. The slowing of the pulse met with on thyroid administration in some cases of tachycardia may be explicable in these terms.

In order, then, to compensate for his hyperexcitable vagus the patient calls in the opposing mechanism. He reaches out, that is to say, towards a new balance between vagus depressor system and sympathetic system. The new balance differs from the old balance of health in one momentous particular: it is a balance between extremes. The daily swing between rest and activity is therefore greatly exaggerated. In accordance as the compensation is complete or incomplete so will the response of the patient to calls for effort be a normal or a limited one.

CHAPTER IV

THE GRAPHIC STUDY OF COMPENSATION IN FUNCTIONAL HEART DISEASE

IF the test of vagus stimulation by deep and sustained inspiration to which we have referred be applied to a patient suffering from functional heart disease it will be found that the phenomenon of slowing and the phenomenon of loss of volume undergo certain variations which at first are of an exceedingly puzzling character.

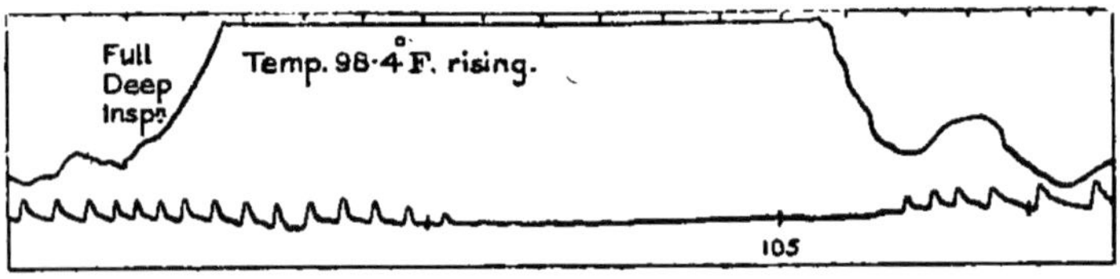

FIG. 13.—Rising Temperature. Pulse disappears on Deep Inspiration.

For example, a patient seen at 10 a.m. presented complete pulsus paradoxus—that is to say, on deep inspiration his pulse entirely disappeared. His temperature was then 98°·4 F. *and was rising* (Fig. 13). Seen at 2 p.m. the pulsus paradoxus was no longer obtainable, but was replaced on deep inspiration by a small-volume *rapid* pulse. The temperature was now 99°·6 F. *and was falling* (Fig. 14). In Figs. 15 and 16 is shown a case in which a short rise of temperature occurred and in which the thyroid was markedly enlarged. At 10 a.m. the temperature was 103° F. One hour and a quarter later the second tracing was taken — temperature still 103° F.; it fell soon after.

In Fig. 17 is shown a tracing from a man with trench fever, taken on the rise of the temperature at 9.30 p.m., 15th January 1918. Temperature was then 101°·5 F. There was a fall of blood

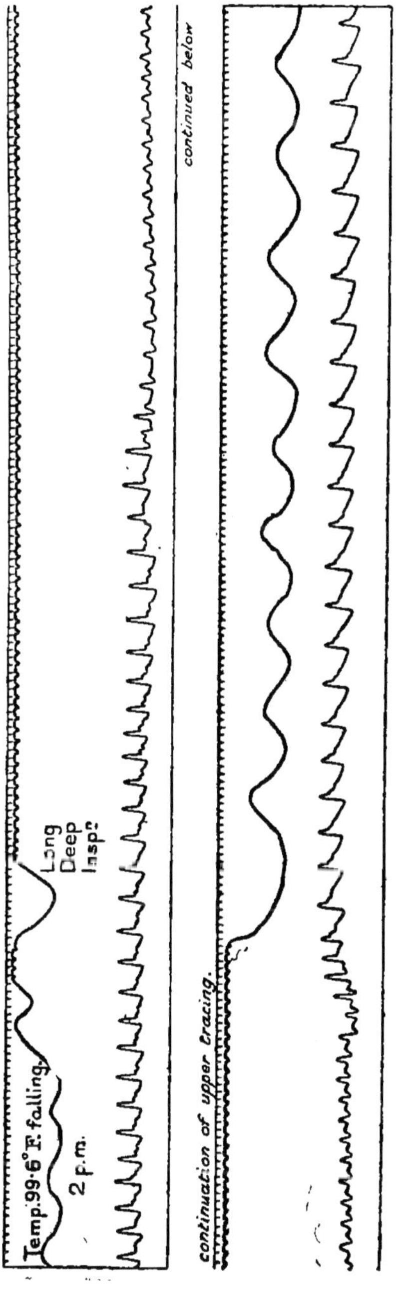

FIG. 14.—Falling Temperature. Pulse no longer disappears on Deep Inspiration.

pressure from 112 systolic before the deep inspiration to 80 systolic during the deep inspiration, which gave rise to a very small pulse which almost amounted to pulsus paradoxus. The patient's temperature rose to 103°·8 F., and at 11.5 p.m.

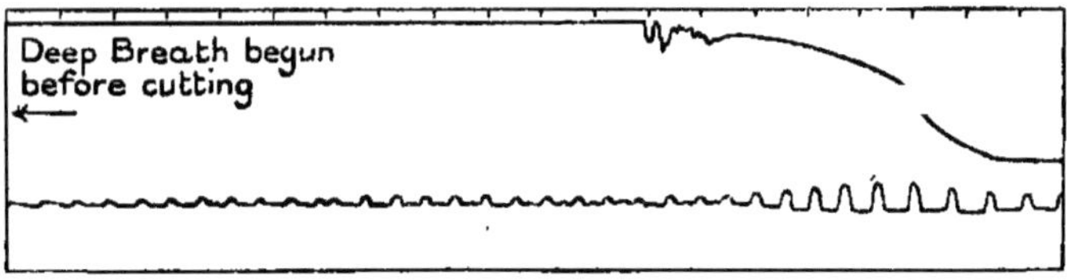

FIG. 15.—Temperature 103° F. Marked Fall in Pulse Volume on Deep Inspiration.

he began to be easier and the temperature to fall. When the temperature was 103°·6 F. another tracing, Fig. 18, was taken; the pulse volume did not now on deep inspiration fall to anything like the same extent. A little later, however, at

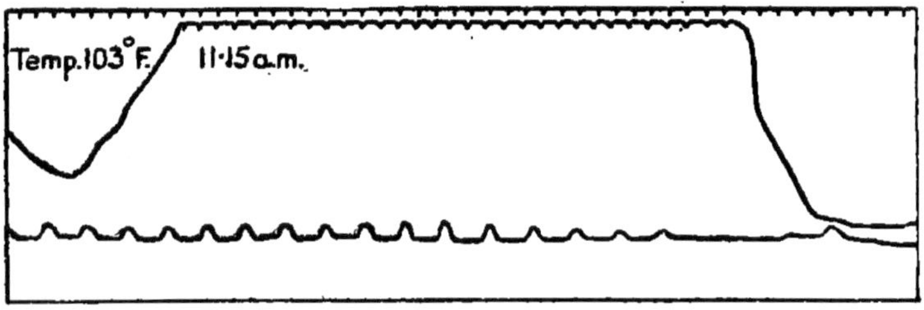

FIG. 16.—Temperature Falling. Fall in Pulse Volume on Deep Inspiration is less well marked.

1.30 p.m., when the temperature was 101° F., it was noted: "Patient begins to feel less well again; pains have returned in shins." A tracing, Fig. 19, was taken, and it was found to resemble Fig. 17 rather closely. At 3 a.m. temperature had risen to 102°·5 F.

These experiences were repeated in other cases, so that it could be said that with a rising temperature in cases of trench fever the loss of pulse volume was more marked, and with a falling temperature it was less marked. In cases of func-

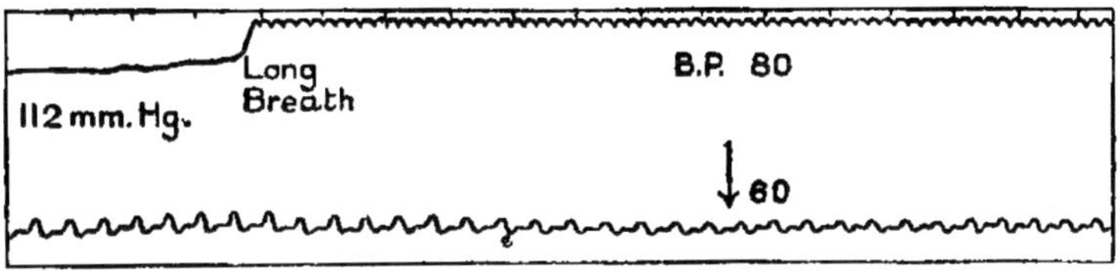

FIG. 17.—Temperature 101°·5 F.

tional heart disease, *e.g.* D.A.H. from rheumatism, when spikes of temperature occurred as they were wont to do, the same rule was found to obtain.

In addition to this observation it was noted that while in some cases the loss of volume was

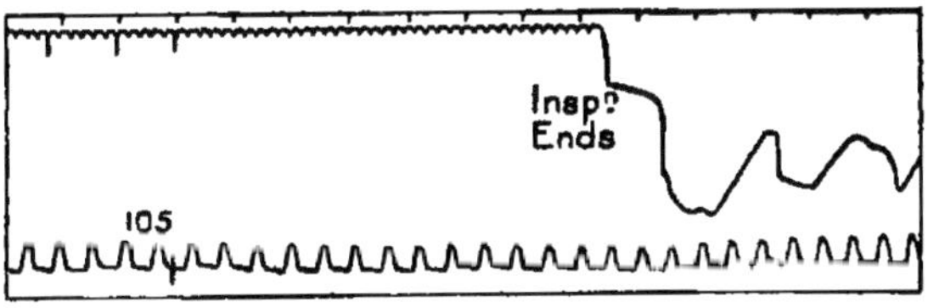

FIG. 18.—Temperature 103°·6 F. Little Fall on Deep Inspiration.

accompanied by slowing, much more frequently it was accompanied by quickening and followed by slowing when the deep inspiration ended (compare Fig. 14 with Fig. 20, which shows a marked fall of volume and a slowing from 70 to 58). Generally speaking, the more marked the fall in volume the more tendency was there for quickening to

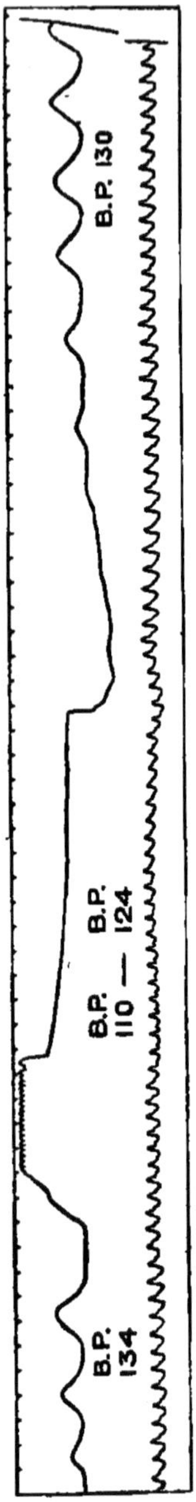

FIG. 19.—Temperature 101° F. (rising for the second time). Fall of Volume on Deep Inspiration.

occur along with it ; indeed, for the most part when slowing occurred the volume tended to augment.

Again, it was found that in some patients a first deep inspiration would produce a sharp fall in volume, while subsequent inspirations produced less, without any change of temperature and indeed within a few minutes.

These three observations, then, may be set side by side :—

(1) Volume fall is most marked during a rising temperature.

(2) The more marked the fall in volume the more tendency is there for the pulse to show quickening, slowing being a delayed phenomenon in these cases, and not occurring till the deep inspiration ends.

(3) In some cases volume fall tends to grow less if rapidly succeeding stimulations of the vagus by deep inspiration are carried out.

It may be added that—

(4) Where only slowing and no volume fall is observed, the slowing is most marked during a rising temperature and also tends to grow less on succeeding stimulations in some instances.

If it be remembered that one of the factors controlling temperature is radiation from the skin and lungs, it will be manifest that a general and marked diastolic state of the hearts and blood lakes making for a general stasis or slowing of the blood flow

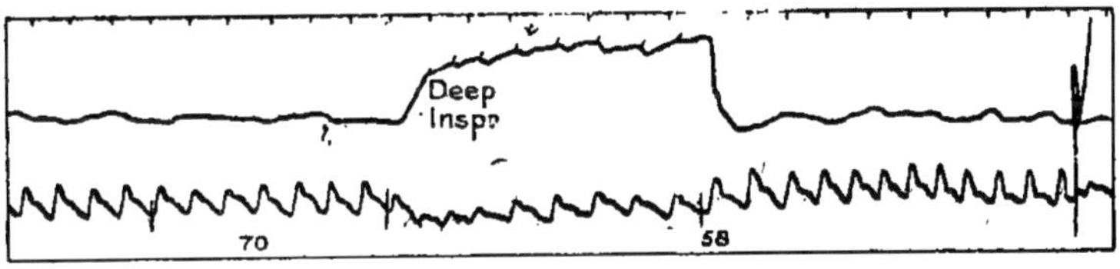

FIG. 20.—Sharp Fall of Pulse Volume and Slowing on Deep Inspiration.

must tend to a rise of temperature. A falling temperature would on this reasoning point to a lowering of vagus depressor irritability. This would explain the coincident phenomena of a rising temperature and a fall of volume at the wrist.

Moreover, the more marked the fall of volume—that is to say, the more excitable the vagus depressor system—the more necessity there must be for sympathetic response or compensation. Up to a point the compensation could be effected by active systoles of the widely opened lakes or hearts (the big diastole giving by a phenomenon of augmentation a larger output of blood at each systole). But beyond that point this augmentation could not occur owing to disturbance of balance between vagus and sympathetic. Thereafter acceleration must be resorted to in order to achieve the result. So that in these instances a stimulation of the vagus mechanism by a deep inspiration will cause *quickening* while it lasts. As the stimulation is gradually lessened, augmentation will be possible again, and long slow beats will appear for a few seconds after the inspiration. In other words, there are two methods of circulatory response to a stimulus both of which are determined by the vagus depressor mechanism—augmentation in which a greater systole succeeds to a greater diastole and the output of blood is thereby increased, and acceleration in which the actual rate of systole is increased. In the normal subject these two mechanisms come into play together during effort. But when the vagus becomes hyper-excitable beyond a certain point too great a burden is imposed on the mechanism of sympathetic response and acceleration has to be dropped—the pulse slows. A still further degree of vagus hyperexcitability, however, so disturbs the balance between vagus and sympathetic that augmentation fails, and then once again acceleration must occur. The rate in this latter case is high and the effect poor; the blood pressure falls markedly.

Finally, each stimulation of the vagus will, as

we have seen, provoke a response in the sympathetic mechanism so that, in cases in which the sympathetic mechanism is averagely active, the vagal phenomena will tend to be more and more obscured by the sympathetic response, *i.e.* the normal condition at each succeeding inspiration. We thus perceive that in cases of functional heart disease of a toxic origin there are three factors always at play :—

(1) The irritability of the vagus depressor determined by the presence or absence of toxin and its amount at any moment.

(2) The degree of response taking place at any moment.

(3) The mental conditions or stimuli acting at the moment.

In these factors is to be found, we believe, the explanation of the notable ups and downs of these patients and their apparently inconsequent changes of temper and mood and physical condition.

CHAPTER V

The Diseases which act directly on the Vagus Depressor Mechanism

UP to this point we have been dealing chiefly with trench fever. But we have been able to establish the fact that there are other diseases which act directly on the vagus depressor mechanism. So far we have established this finding for "rheumatism," "rheumatoid arthritis," "acute rheumatism," and a few other conditions. That these conditions—"rheumatism" especially, by which is meant the condition of pains and aches, so indefinite in ætiology so definite in character, which abounds in this country—play a part in the ætiology of functional heart diseases is not open to serious dispute. Figs. 21 and 22 illustrate what we mean, and other tracings are given later in the text.

We suggest that in these diseases, as in trench fever, a toxin acts upon the vagus depressor mechanism, increasing its irritability, as can be shown. The exact nature of the toxin we do not

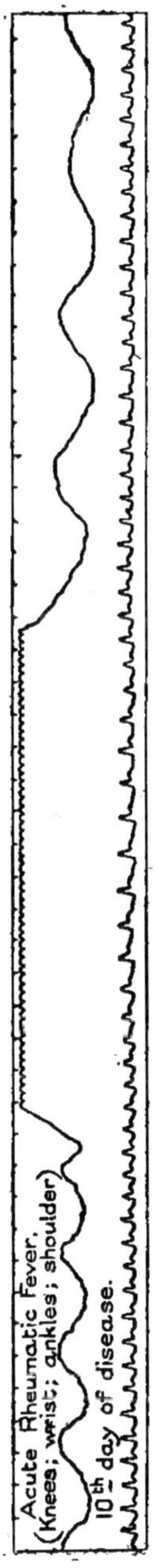

FIG. 21.—Note marked Slowing on Deep Inspiration.

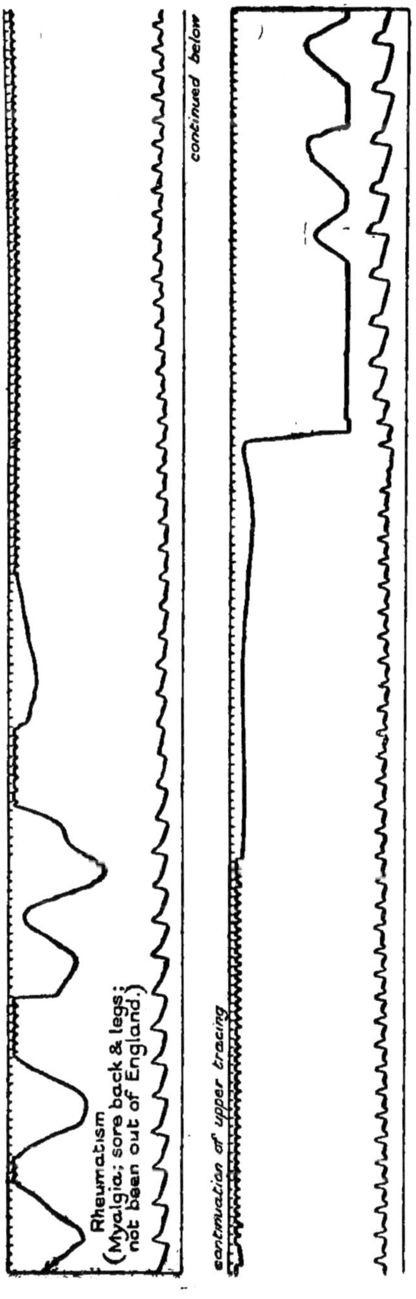

FIG. 22.—Note marked Volume Fall and Quickening on Deep Inspiration. Slowing follows the end of the Inspiration.

know. The mechanism of the production of functional heart disease in these states is therefore the same as the mechanism of its production in trench fever.

The Toxic Origin of Functional Heart Disease.—That trench fever and rheumatism are the forerunners of functional heart disease there is no doubt. Of a series of 66 cases seen at Fulham Military Hospital who had served at home or in France only, 30 had had rheumatism or rheumatic fever before joining, while 32 had had some form of pyrexia on service. The remainder were gas cases. These vague pyrexias of service are nearly certainly trench fever as has been abundantly proved by Major Byam's work at Hampstead and the work of the Trench Fever Commission in France.

A subsequent series of 72 cases at Mount Vernon Hospital for the Study of D.A.H. showed 21 with rheumatism and rheumatic fever before joining, and 38 with vague fevers in France classed as rheumatism, myalgia, trench fever, and so on. Mackenzie, Lewis, MacIlwaine, and others have emphasized the toxic origin of many cases of functional heart disease.

Our investigations lead us to suppose that many other diseases produce functional heart disease as a sequel, and we have recently proved this in dysentery, Kala-azar, malaria, and other tropical conditions; but as so many cases can be definitely put down to rheumatism and its allies we do not propose to enter further into this aspect of the question, leaving consideration of it to other investigators.

CHAPTER VI

The Nature of the Temperature Curve encountered in Functional Heart Disease

THE prevalent view that in cases of functional heart disease the temperature remains normal is certainly erroneous. A very large number of investigations have shown us that in these cases the normal daily swing of the temperature is often greatly exaggerated, and further, that so-called "spikes" of temperature are liable to occur from time to time without apparent cause.

Some Typical Cases.—Fig. 23 shows a spike in a man diagnosed as functional heart disease and admitted to Mount Vernon Hospital, July 1917, for soldiers' heart. The patient had an attack of trench fever in 1916, and thereafter began to feel giddy and breathless and very exhausted. His limbs ached and he could not walk. He stated on admission that he suffered from fatigue, drowsiness, shortness of breath, pains over the præcordium, weakness of the legs, and giddiness. He looked pale and ill, had cold, blue, clammy hands. Heart was not en-

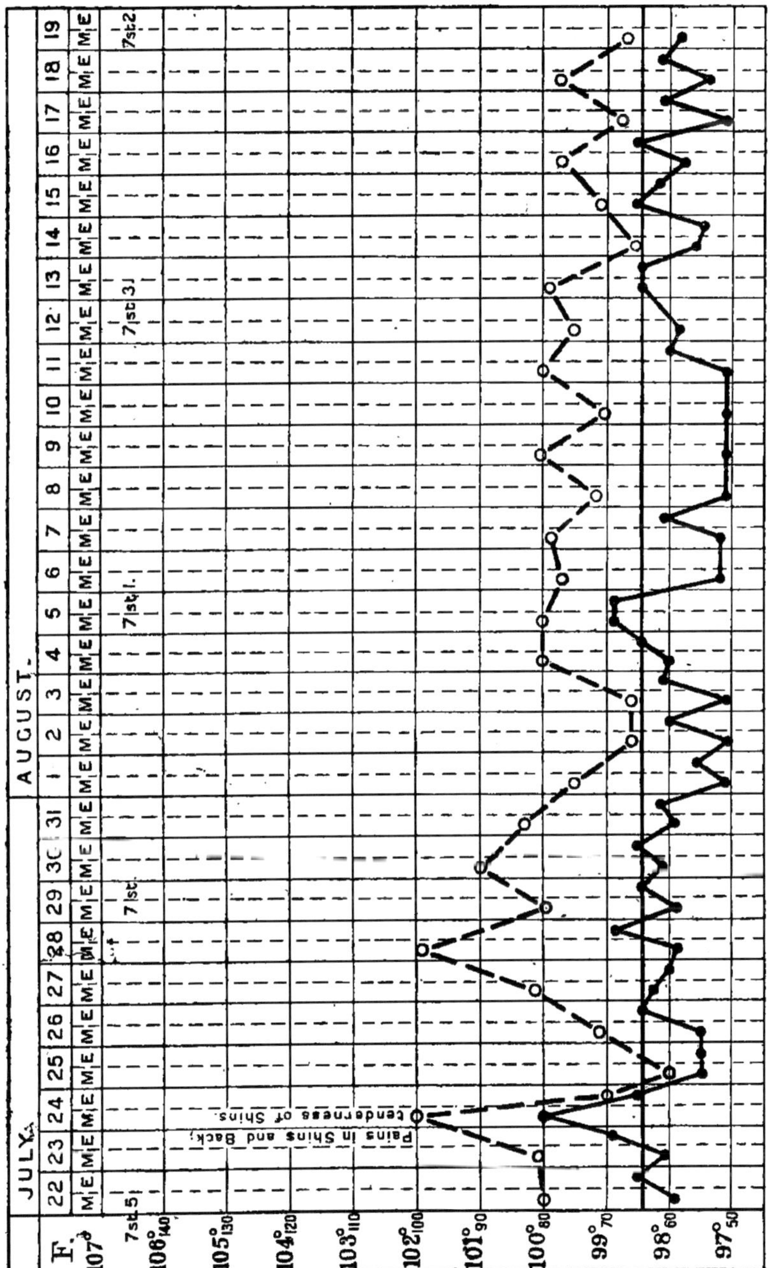

FIG. 23.—D.A.H. and Trench Fever. Pulse and Temperature during Spike of Fever.

larged, but a systolic murmur was heard at the apex. He was nervous and showed marked tremor. There was tenderness over the præcordium.

Fig. 24 shows a spike in a man diagnosed as functional heart disease and admitted to Mount Vernon Hospital, July 1917. He was a case of rheumatism, which he contracted on service in March 1917. Field Card Report was " pain in back and head. T. 98, pulse 74. Apex beat in fifth space, just external to nipple line. Systolic murmur at apex. Premature beats fairly frequently. Abnormal acceleration of the heart rate on exertion." Diagnoses of D.A.H., V.D.H., rheumatism, myalgia, and trench fever were made at different times in this case. The man complained of shortness of breath, shakiness and exhaustion, slight giddiness, and some leg pains. He had præcordial hyperalgesia, a slightly dilated heart, and a loud systolic murmur.

Figs. 25 and 26 illustrate the same points, and are all from cases of functional disease of the heart diagnosed as such by many specialist observers.

Variations of Temperature, Swings, and Spikes are characteristic of Functional Heart Disease. — It is clear, then, that " swings " of temperature and " spikes " are characteristic of functional heart diseases, and that they have frequently been missed because they have not been looked for with suffi-

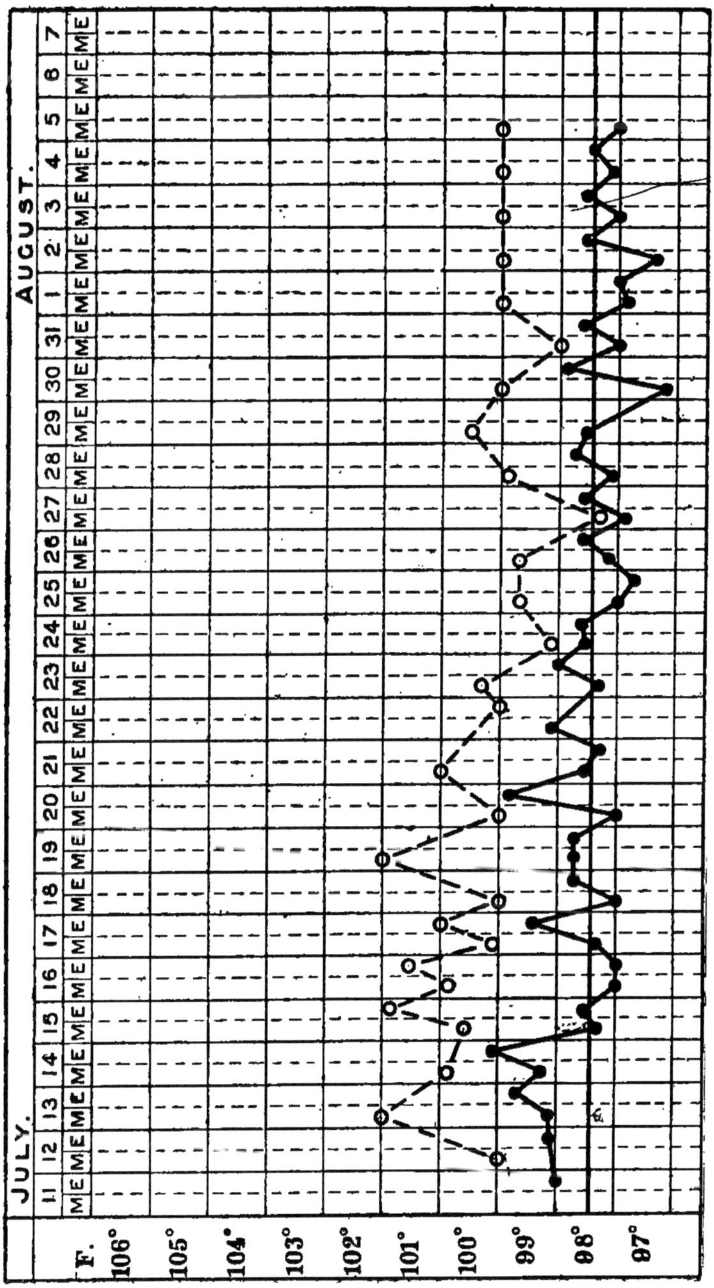

FIG. 24.—D.A.H. and Rheumatism. Illustrating Relation of Pulse to Temperature during Spike of Fever. (Pulse: broken line. Temperature: continuous dark line.)

cient care. We have already suggested that in the circumstance of an irritable vagus depressor mechanism an explanation of this daily swing can be found.

As is universally accepted, the temperature tends to be lowest in the morning normally and to be highest in the evening—about 10 p.m. The

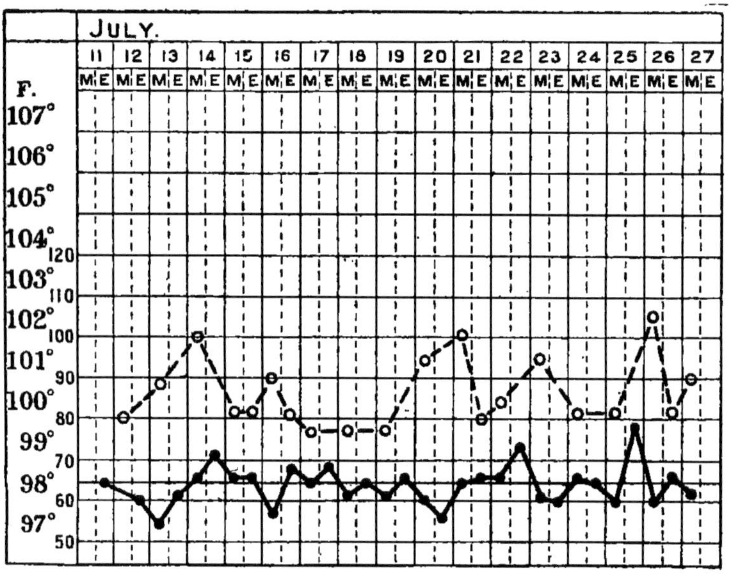

FIG. 25.—D.A.H. Pulse and Temperature.

swing is generally put at about 1 degree. That is to say, that at the time the subject is rested and ready to be active his temperature is low, while when he has reacted and is ready to rest his temperature is high. In other words, when his reacting or sympathetic mechanism is strong his temperature is low, while when his resting or vagus

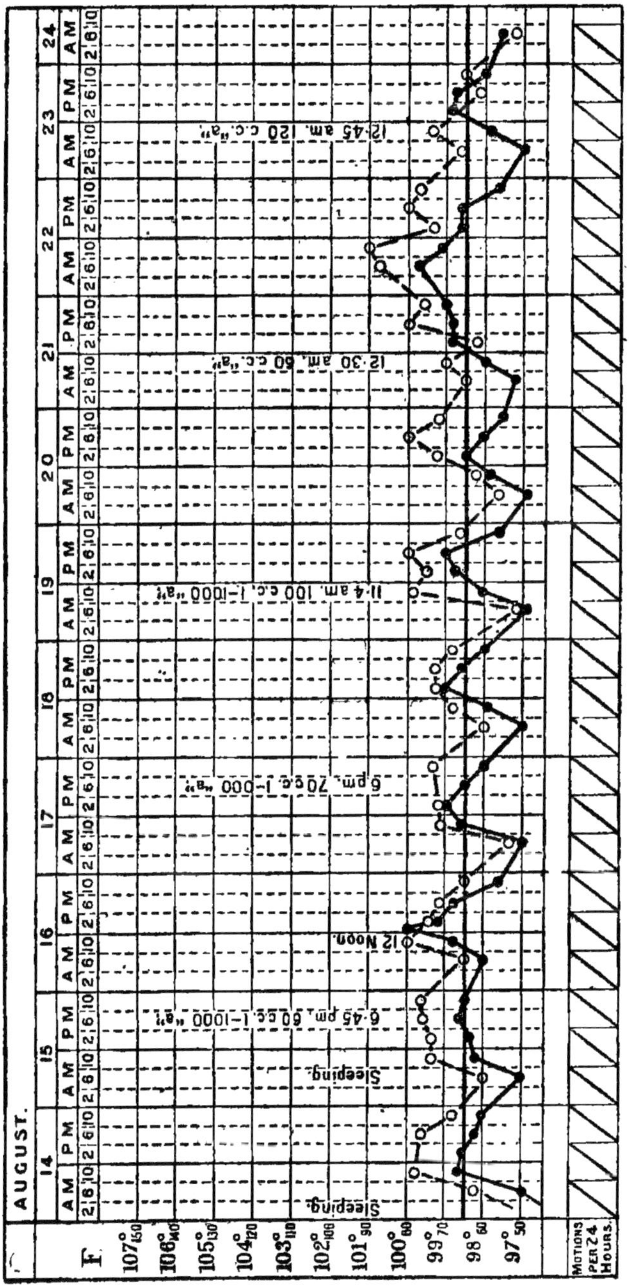

FIG. 26.—D.A.H., Pulse and Temperature.

depressor mechanism is strong his temperature tends to rise.

The temperature then seems to tend to rise as the vagus depressor mechanism becomes more excitable, and to fall as the sympathetic mechanism becomes more excitable. Undoubtedly temperature depends on the relation of heat generated to heat lost. It is a matter of universal knowledge that even the most severe muscular exertion does not raise the skin or oral temperature to any notable extent, so that, evidently, provided the radiation system is acting normally the amount of heat generated does not greatly signify.

The rectal temperature is raised during effort. Major Wm. Byam informs us that at the end of a football match he took rectal temperatures of players, and all were raised, some to 105° F.

The Vagus Depressor Mechanism is the Radiator System.—As we have already stated, the vagus depressor mechanism opens the blood lakes or hearts and tends to hold them in diastole. These lakes are the heart itself (right and left), the pulmonary blood lake (see *Hearts of Man*), the abdominal blood lake, and the peripheral or skin blood lake. This latter, from its position, is evidently the chief radiator of the body, because in it a large quantity of blood is spread over a large area in close apposition to the air, and, thanks to evaporation of sweat, in the best conditions for cooling. The same applies to the pulmonary blood lake in lesser degree, the heat lost by the breathing representing an important amount.

Cooling evidently will depend on three factors :—

1. The rate of blood flow in the radiators skin lake, and pulmonary lake.
2. The bulk of blood, relative to the total blood bulk, exposed in these lakes.
3. The activity of sweating.

Now it is clear that *up to a point* a hyperexcitable condition of the vagus depressor mechanism will result in an increased bulk of blood being exposed in the skin and lungs because these lakes will be widely opened—so-called vaso-dilatation. Moreover, the rate of blood flow will be sufficient, because full strong systoles will follow the deep diastoles.

Beyond this point, however, the picture will change. As the vagus depressor system becomes still more excitable the blood lakes will open wider and the sympathetic response in augmentation and acceleration will become less and less adequate to meet this great "pull." The result must be :—

1. A lessened bulk of blood being exposed in the skin and lungs, because now the widely opened abdominal lake will hold so large an amount of the blood (Fig. 27).
2. The rate of blood flow will be diminished owing to the grip of the vagus depressor upon the lakes exceeding in strength the response of the sympathetic

mechanism—that is to say, owing to the weakening of motor force of the circulation stasis of blood will occur in the lakes (a stasis manifested in actual life by a cyanosis of the skin).

During lesser degrees of vagus depressor hyperexcitability, then, the temperature will tend to be subnormal owing to increased cooling; during greater degrees of vagus depressor hyperexcitability it will tend to rise above normal with some evidence of capillary stasis or congestion.

So we obtain the rule :—

Normal vagus depressor excitability means normal temperature; somewhat greater than normal vagus depressor excitability means subnormal temperature; much greater than normal vagus depressor excitability means a rise of temperature above normal.

Vagus Excitability determines Temperature Swing.— Consequently in patients with a hyperexcitable vagus depressor mechanism we should expect a daily swing from subnormal to supernormal— that is, in the evening, when the reaction mechanism or sympathetic is tired, and so less capable of adequate response, we should expect slight rises of temperature, say to 99° F.; in the morning, when the reaction mechanism or sympathetic is refreshed and restored and so more capable of adequate response, we should expect subnormal temperatures, *e.g.* 96° F., 97° F., or 98° F.

This is exactly what we get in cases of functional heart disease.

Further, any fresh outpouring of toxin by increasing vagus hyper-excitability would cause a "spike" of temperature.

The sympathetic system—the system of response—must answer the call of the vagus depressor mechanism, no matter whether the latter be less or more excitable. Therefore if the sympathetic system, in process of compensation, becomes as hyper-excitable as the hyper-excitable vagus depressor the "swing" of temperature will stop, or rather return to the normal—about 1 degree between night and morning. In functional heart disease 2 and 3 degrees of a swing is a common feature.

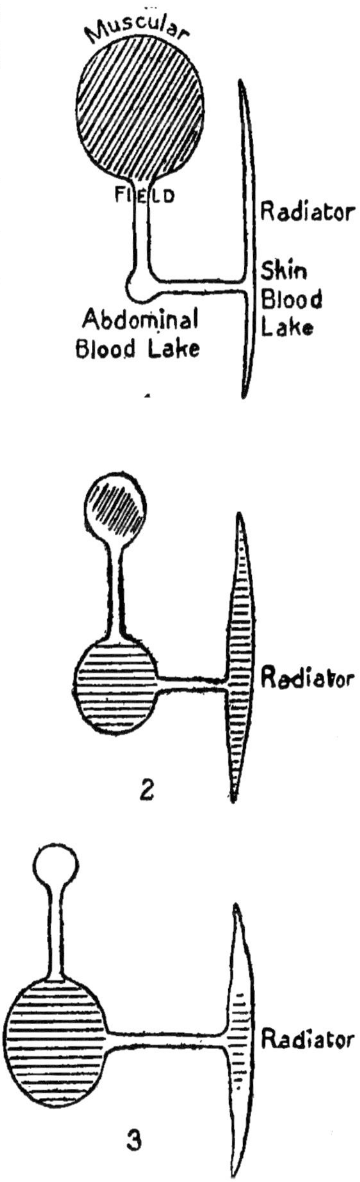

FIG. 27.—Illustrates how the Radiator of the Skin may be emptied when blood is gathered in mesenteric lake and stasis occurs.

Spikes of Temperature are Toxic in Origin.—A study of the "spikes" of temperature in this respect is most interesting. On the "rise" the patient will be seen to be pale and shivery—if the attack is severe he may be deadly pale and may even faint. Cold sweats occur. When the fastigium is reached the skin becomes a dusky red, signifying the growing adequacy of sympathetic response to the vagus depressor "pull." The stasis is evident, because the lips are cyanotic, the skin tending to blueness, the eyes suffused. The skin feels hot, and owing to the heat sweat is evaporated very quickly. Then as the sympathetic response becomes more adequate the temperature begins to fall, the dusky colour gives place to a fresh red, the stasis disappears, the skin is full of blood, and warm sweats occur.

We have already pointed out that during the rise of temperature deep inspiration produces a marked loss of pulse volume with, in severe cases, a rapid pulse; during the fall of temperature this phenomenon is either much modified or has entirely disappeared. Consequently it would seem that the fall of temperature here occurs because the output of toxin has been stopped, and so the hyperexcitable state of the vagus depressor mechanism reduced rather than because the response of the sympathetic mechanism has undergone a sudden increase.

The daily swing of 2 or 3 degrees in functional

heart disease is therefore probably not immediately toxic in origin—that is to say, it is determined by the ordinary conditions of living acting upon a vagus depressor system rendered somewhat hyperexcitable by a toxin; but the "spike" would seem to be immediately toxic and due to a new outpouring of toxin over and above the usual amount in circulation in the blood.

CHAPTER VII

Pulse Rate in Functional Heart Disease

PROBABLY no subject has received closer study by more competent observers than that of pulse rate in functional heart disease. The most recent observations are those of Lewis and his fellow-workers at Mount Vernon (of whom one of the writers was one). Lewis thus states his view (Report to Medical Research Committee):—

"When the patients are completely rested, the average heart rate is about 85 per minute in unselected cases. In sleep the rates are for the most part normal. In patients who are up and about the average is higher, being from 90 to 100 to the minute. Exceptionally, patients present rates of 120 or 130 per minute in the same circumstances, and very rarely the same rates may continue for weeks while the patients are in bed.

"As a rule it may be said that the rates approach more closely the rates of health the more rigidly responses to effort and emotion are eliminated. It is clear that the excessive rates found in the majority of these subjects are conditioned by exaggerated response to natural stimuli (such as effort and emotion)."

These views we accept, and we desire to emphasize the fact that excessive rates are conditioned by exaggerated responses to effort or emotion—that is to say, to stimuli.

We have already expressed and explained our view that the vagus depressor system is activated by every stimulus reaching the individual. This system determines the subsequent reaction which, in its essence, is a pressor reaction having as its object the charging of the muscular field with blood derived from the blood lakes or hearts. In other language, the sympathetic system closes the hearts by throwing them, through the instrumentality of a series of increasingly complete systoles (followed in each instance by increasingly incomplete diastoles), into the condition of plus-systole and so expels a mass of contained blood. This mass is thus driven into the muscles (and brain), there being no other place for it to go.

Pressor Effects are obtained normally by Augmentation and then by Acceleration.—It is a matter of experience that the heart beats more strongly during effort or excitement, and so is said to "thump." The mechanism of this augmentation is evident the moment it is remembered that, normally, an increased diastole determines a larger output of blood at the following systole—or, in other words, that the first response of the sympathetic to vagus depressor action is a big systole. That is to say, vagus depressor action in prolonging diastole calls for stronger systolic efforts or "augmentation." Acceleration can be added as an extra help if necessary. Acceleration, however, is a purely sympathetic phenomenon and represents an increase in the frequency of systole. This is the normal mechanism. If, however, the vagus becomes hyperexcitable beyond a certain point, acceleration and augmentation can no longer be supplied by the sympathetic and acceleration is dropped. The result is a slow pulse with augmented beats, but even this may fail if further vagus excitability occurs. Then again acceleration must occur.

In Disease, if Augmentation fails, Acceleration of an extreme type becomes necessary.—We have already touched upon this in considering the graphic records of pulses (Chapter IV.). It is clear that when the vagus depressor mechanism reaches a certain degree of excitability the diastolic state resulting will be so great and the hearts will be so actively held in diastole that augmentation sufficiently powerful to produce the necessary pressor effects will be impossible; the mechanism of reaction, *i.e.* the sympathetic mechanism, will in these cases produce acceleration again with the object of increasing the response and so preventing collapse and death.

We have already seen from our tracings (Figs. 14 and 22) that when deep inspiration produces a marked fall of pulse volume it also, as a rule, produces a marked quickening of the pulse—the slowing and pure augmentation coming later at the end of the deep inspiration when the excitation of the vagus depressor is suspended. This quickening, then, is a direct response to an extreme degree of vagus depressor hyperexcitability. The more excitable the vagus depressor mechanism the more will this quickening be evidenced, the less excitable the vagus depressor mechanism the less will it be evidenced. There are thus the following stages :—

1. *Normal Vagus.*—Stimulus causes vagus pull with augmentation, acceleration (quick pulse), and plus-systole and a response in excess of the pull. Effort is possible.
2. *Slightly Excitable Vagus.*—The same: only pulse will be more rapid than normal.
3. *Hyperexcitable Vagus.*—Stimulus causes vagus pull with only augmentation (slow pulse). Acceleration has to be dropped and response is weak and usually inadequate. Less plus-systole achieved.
4. *More Hyperexcitable Vagus.*—Augmentation becomes impossible owing to upset of balance between vagus and sympathetic. Only acceleration remains. Stimulus causes therefore a very rapid pulse with fall of blood presssure and no plus-systole. Effort impossible.

The Palpitation complained of by Patients with Functional Heart Disease is Augmentation with Acceleration, because in these cases a measure of compensation has been established. But they are responding too violently to light Stimuli.—We thus arrive at once at an explanation of "palpitation" of which Lewis writes :—

"Palpitation is a very frequent complaint . . . is an expression of rapid and vigorous heart action ; it may be maintained under all conditions ; more commonly it is present or severe chiefly *during* exercise or under emotion. Meakins and Gunson have clearly established its relation to excessive heart rate in patients in whom it is provoked by exercise ; for it is no longer felt after the rate has declined to a certain point. When the decline is gradual, palpitation disappears gradually ; when, as may happen, there is an abrupt decline of pulse rate, there is a simultaneous and abrupt relief from the sensation. Palpitation of this kind calls for no treatment in itself. Its significance is that of the associated high pulse rate."

We need not labour this point. It is evident. The rapid pulse is merely a good, strong reaction to a somewhat excitable vagus (see 2, page 71).

The Rapid Pulse of Functional Heart Disease is therefore determined by Vagus Depressor Excitability.—It will be immediately objected to the foregoing that if it be true that vagus depressor hyperexcitability accounts for the rapid pulse rate in functional heart disease, atropine, which inhibits vagal endings, should slow the pulse in these cases and should not quicken it. Indeed, Lewis and Cotton and Rapport, as the result of giving $\frac{1}{500}$ grain atropine per stone of body weight intravenously (*i.e.* $\frac{1}{41}$ grain to a 12-stone man), came to the conclusion that—

"The effect of atropine upon the heart rate in patient and control is identical in its degree. It is to be concluded, therefore, that vagal tone is unaltered and that a reduction of vagal tone is not responsible for raised cardiac rate in these patients."

In order to comprehend the fallacy of this reasoning it is necessary to realize that augmentation is a sympathetic response to a vagal pull. It is thus in a sense a joint vagal and sympathetic phenomenon. In response to a stimulus the vagus depressor acts by increasing diastole: the subsequent systole is augmented in force to counterbalance this. As the reaction goes on, the lakes and heart go into plus-systole—*i.e.* diastolize less, but the augmentor action continues.

Therefore any drug which inhibits the vagus depressor mechanism prevents augmentation by removing part of the mechanism necessary to its accomplishment.

Now $\frac{1}{41}$ grain atropine intravenously is a very large dose, and in Lewis's seven cases caused an average rise of pulse rate of 26 beats per minute. In short, the vagus depressor mechanism was inhibited and so part of the mechanism necessary to the accomplishment of augmentation removed.

Acceleration remained the only means of responding to a call for effort (with vagi cut adrenalin or sympathetic stimulation produces only acceleration : Schäfer).

It appeared to us, therefore, that the proper test of vagus depressor hyperexcitability was to give a dose of atropine of a much smaller amount, so as, if possible, to convert our hyperexcitable vagus depressor into a vagus depressor of normal excitability still capable of reacting well to stimuli by increasing diastole, yet no longer so active as to render augmentation insufficient to meet the needs of the moment. We accordingly gave $\frac{1}{200}$ grain intravenously to five cases with D.A.H. The graphic records are appended (Fig. 28). In four cases marked slowing occurred, in one slowing was only 4 beats and was followed by a subsequent quickening—*but the pulse rate in this latter case to begin with was only* 68.

The figures are :—

(*a*) 105 slowed to 85 in 4 minutes.
(*b*) 68 ,, ,, 64 in 1½ ,,
(*c*) 98 ,, ,, 65 in 5 ,,
(*d*) 85 ,, ,, 56 in 1½ ,,
(*e*) 108 ,, ,, 85 in 4 ,,

Thus of the four with pulses above 80 the average rate before atropine was 99 and the average slowing 29 beats after it.

The patient with a pulse rate of 68 slowed only to 64.

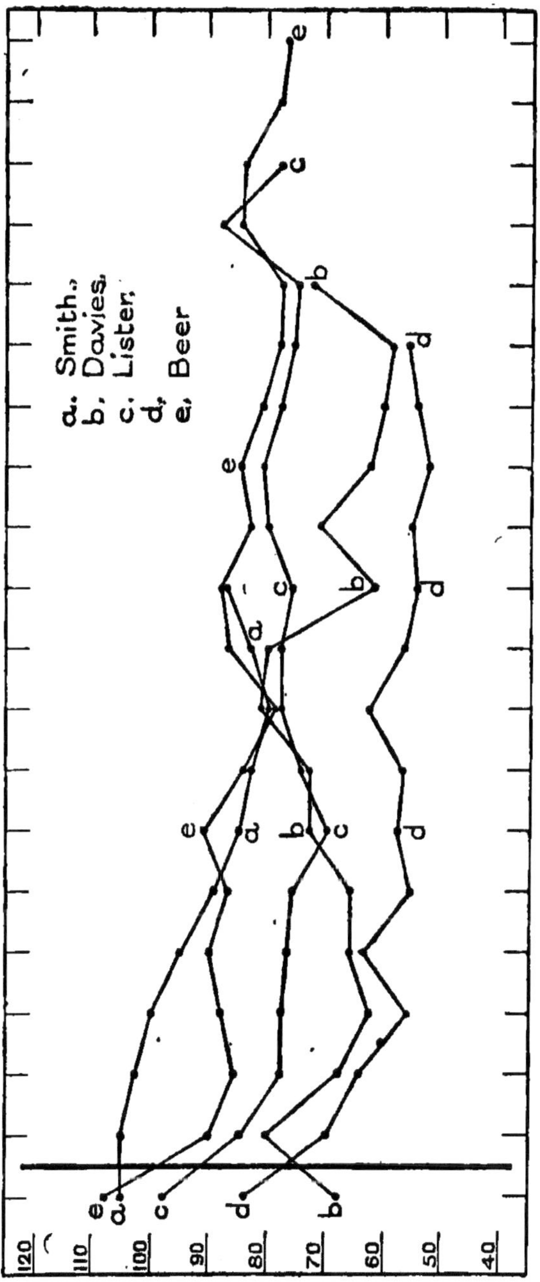

FIG. 28.—Graphic Records of Pulse Rate after a Dose of $\frac{1}{200}$ grain Atropine intravenously. Tracings taken with polygraph. The perpendicular line shows point of injection. Note the fall in rate in all cases except "b."

We therefore see that to give maximal doses of atropine and so to abolish the possibility of augmentation is to make acceleration a certainty, no matter whether the vagus is normal or hyperexcitable. It is only when minimal doses are given and a hyperexcitable vagus reduced to a lower degree of excitement that we gain real knowledge. Then, augmentation being increased in pressor effectiveness, acceleration is no longer necessary and the pulse rate at once falls.

Incidentally this disposes of the idea that atropine in small doses acts as a vagus irritant, because, were that true, the patient with the slow pulse, 68, would have slowed just as the other patients did. In his failure to slow to any extent and his tendency, on the contrary, to quicken, we see an indication that atropine does inhibit the vagus depressor mechanism even in the smallest doses. If this mechanism is normal, "release" occurs with small doses, because the mechanism necessary to the accomplishment of augmentation is weakened by the small doses; if the mechanism is hyperexcitable, slowing occurs because augmentation is strengthened. In other words, both abnormal weakness and abnormal strength of the vagus depressor mechanism interfere with the process of augmentation, the former by preventing sufficient diastole and the latter by preventing sufficient systole. In both these cases acceleration thus becomes necessary to achieve the needful pressor effects. We have discussed this fully above.

Atropine in Large Doses by abolishing Augmentation causes Acceleration.—This conclusion is well illustrated in Figs. 29, 30, and 31. In the first and second of these (29 and 30), slowing and augmen-

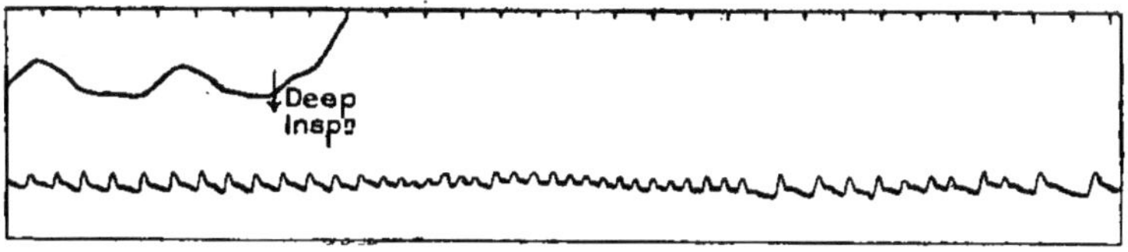

Before Atropine.

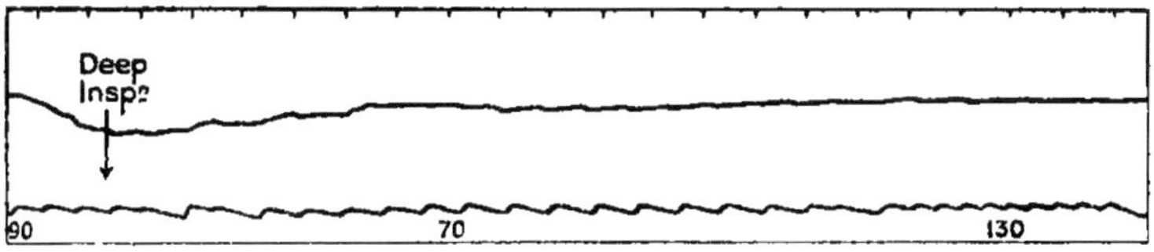

Before Atropine.

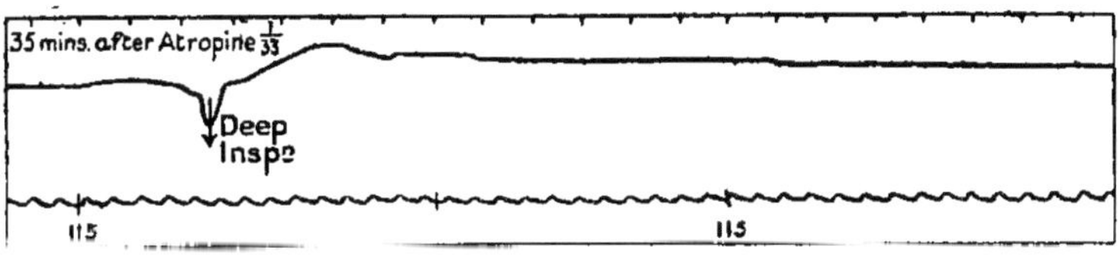

After Atropine.

FIGS. 29, 30, and 31.—Effect of Atropine on a Pulse, showing both slowing and quickening on deep inspiration.

tation with "breaks" of acceleration are shown as the result of deep inspiration, *i.e.* of vagus stimulation. In the third (31), after $\frac{1}{33}$ grain of atropine, "release" of 25 beats has taken place and the vagus is no longer excitable—acceleration has replaced augmentation throughout the whole pulse picture.

Lewis's conclusion, then, that "vagal tone is unaltered" in functional heart disease would not seem to be justified, though we may agree with him that "a *reduction* of vagal tone is not responsible for raised cardiac rate in these patients." (The italics are ours.)

The Return of the Pulse after Effort is Rapid or Slow in Functional Heart Disease according as the Vagus is less or more Hyperexcitable.—It follows from the above that if the vagus is only slightly hyperexcitable, "return of the pulse" after effort will be sudden and quick—in other words, acceleration will rapidly give place to augmentation, which will be a good and sufficient response in the circumstances. The end of effort represents the end of a reaction, and so the swing back from that reaction to rest. If the vagus is very hyperexcitable, on the other hand acceleration will be necessary even after effort to counteract the strong diastolic pull, and consequently will be kept up—though at a constantly declining level — until gradually augmentation may be established. Thereafter augmentation also will die away and the normal resting state be resumed.

Therefore in very hyperexcitable vagus depressor states the pulse will run up above the usual height on effort and will return to normal more slowly than usual. In less hyperexcitable vagus depressor states the exact opposite will occur. The pulse will not rise so high nor yet return so slowly, because the pull into diastole will not be so severe either at the beginning or at the end of effort.

In an atropinized subject there will be a greatly reduced vagal pull at the beginning of effort, and

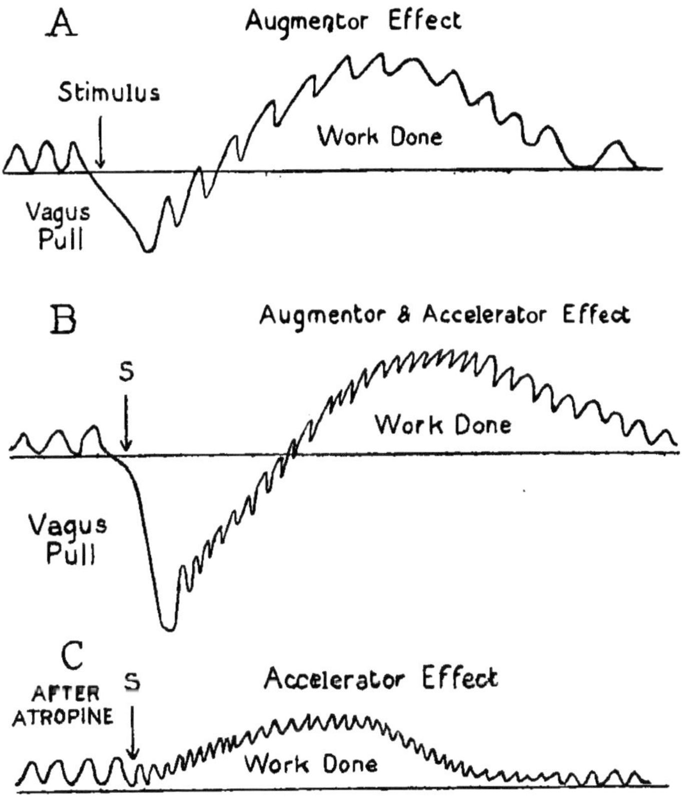

FIGS. 32, 33, and 34.—Pressor Efforts in response to Stimuli varying with state of vagus excitability.

so very little opportunity of augmented beating (*i.e.* more powerful systoles) will occur. The lakes and heart will not therefore tend to pass into plus-systole, but will merely show an accelerated rate of beating. The differences between these efforts are shown diagrammatically (Figs. 32, 33, and 34).

In the first of the figures (Fig. 32) the vagus depressor pulls normally and an easy response takes place, each succeeding systole being of longer duration than the preceding one, so that the lakes are closed and the pressor effect got without acceleration.

In the second (Fig. 33), the vagus pulls more violently, and the pressor effect required is only got by means of acceleration and augmentation (" palpitation ").

In the third (Fig. 34), the pressor effect is obtained only by most extreme acceleration (the vagus being inhibited by atropine)—a strain upon the sympathetic mechanism which could not long be endured.

Any increase of vagus hyperexcitability beyond Fig. 33 will prevent the accomplishment of effort. Acceleration will require to be dropped altogether, giving a slow pulse. A still further hyperexcitability will so upset the relations of vagus and sympathetic that the augmentation mechanism will break down. Blood pressure will fall, and an extremely rapid, very low tension pulse be met with. (See discussion above.)

CHAPTER VIII

BREATHLESSNESS

IF a very close study of respiratory phenomena be made, it will be found that there are two distinct types of breathing, which one of the writers in *The Hearts of Man* has called reaction breathing and rest breathing.

Rest Breathing is the normal mechanism of respiration, the main object of which is oxygenation of the blood. It is chiefly carried out by the diaphragm, of which the motor nerve is the phrenic. The *afferent* or " sensory " nerve of diaphragmatic or rest breathing is the vagus.

Reaction Breathing is the mechanism of respiration designed to secure, or rather assist, pressor effects in periods of effort of one sort or another. Its main object is therefore not oxygenation. It is carried on by the so-called extraordinary muscles of respiration, notably the serratus magnus, the recti and abdominal wall muscles, *and the glottis*. The diaphragm plays little or no part in it. Its motor nerve supply consists of the nerves to the muscles concerned. The sympathetic system acts as its sensory supply. (Sherrington showed that stimulation of the sympathetic caused contraction of the abdominal wall muscles.) The shapes of the chest in these two types of breathing are figured (Figs. 35 and 36).

The Muscular Mechanism of Reaction Breathing.—

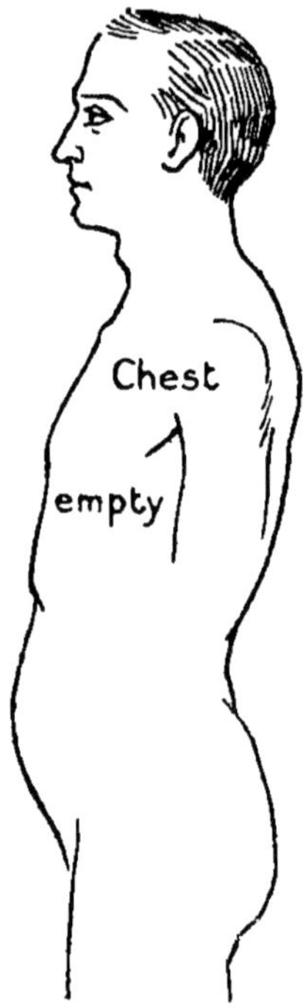

FIG. 35.—Shape of Chest and Abdomen in Rest Breathing.

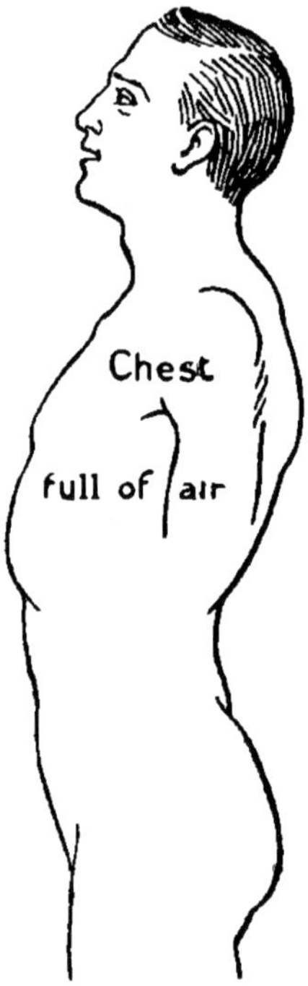

FIG. 36.—Shape of Chest and Abdomen in Reaction Breathing.

The muscular mechanism of reaction breathing reduced to its simplest form is a mechanism whereby, the glottis being closed, the muscles of the abdominal wall contract on the abdominal contents, and acting like the thrust of a syringe drive blood out of the mesenteric lake and also out of the pulmonary lake into the muscular field and brain. So long as the glottis is held shut this muscular thrust will be very powerful, *and the contained air in the chest will serve as a pneumatic buffer between the thrusting muscles and the expelled blood.* It will be found that even during the simplest efforts—close thinking, speaking, listening intently, and so on—the glottis is closed and a slight tightening of the abdominal muscles occurs. These actions have been recorded graphically, and tracings showing them will be found in *The*

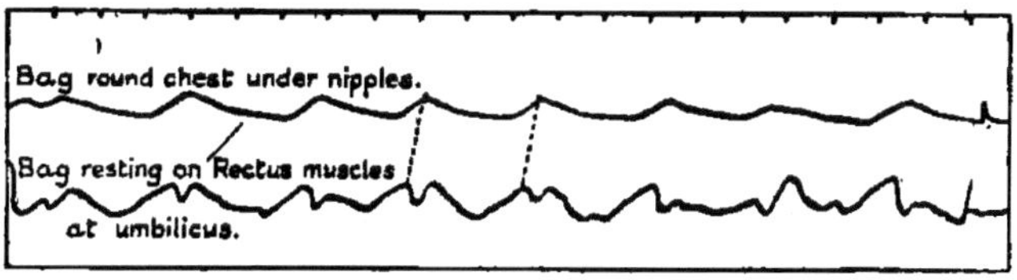

FIG. 37.—Note twitch of rectus at each inspiration.

Hearts of Man. (Fig. 37 shows the twitch of the rectus at each inspiration in a case of fever.)

It is clear, therefore, that the more air the lungs contain at the moment the glottis closes and the thrust of the abdominal muscles begins, the more effective that thrust will be in driving blood out into the muscular field (and brain). In other words, the contained air is like a lever and gives "purchase" to the abdominal muscles so that they can effectively assist in expelling blood.

The Voluntary Muscles and the Hearts.—But we have already spoken of the production of pressor effects in terms of the action of the sympathetic in responding to the vagus depressor mechanism by shutting the blood lakes. Clearly this muscular mechanism is an adjuvant to that mechanism of arterioles of which the " hearts " are made up. And, as we would expect and have seen, the muscular mechanism is controlled afferently by the sympathetic, which also produces the plus-systole of the " hearts."

The Vagus Depressor determines the Respiratory Response to Effort just as it determines the Circulatory Response.—We have seen, however, that the pressor response to effort so far as pure circulatory phenomena are concerned is determined in the first instance by the pull of the vagus depressor in reaction to particular stimuli. This pull imposes the necessity of making a response on the sympathetic, and an " augmentor " effect results which affords the needful raising of pressure without in the majority of instances of small efforts much or any acceleration.

Are we able in a study of the respiratory phenomena of effort to discover any analogous action of the vagus depressor? Undoubtedly we are. The vagus being the afferent nerve of diaphragmatic respiration will tend when excited to induce a contraction of that muscle, and thus will tend to draw air into the chest—the familiar " gasp " of surprise, or deeper inspiration of beginning effort.

But this drawing of air into the chest at once augments the force of reaction breathing if that should follow immediately after the vagal effect, and secures that a greater pressor effect will be produced by the abdominal muscles in their contraction.

In carrying out any effort, then, a preliminary vagus pull will be of marked advantage, provided that the excitability of the vagus depressor system is not of too extreme a degree—*that is to say, provided the vagus is not so irritable that the glottis cannot be held shut* to resist the subsequent thrust of the abdominal muscles and give the pneumatic buffer effect.

It was long ago observed by Hering and Brewer that if the trachea was plugged at the end of inspiration the succeeding expiration was enormously prolonged and strengthened and *an immediate relaxation of the diaphragm occurred*—*i.e.* reaction breathing began. We have only to imagine a condition of vagus excitability so great that this relaxation of the diaphragm would not occur *and the glottis thus not be able to be held shut*, to perceive that in hyperexcitable vagus states the normal augmentor mechanism might fail to produce the pressor effect required and in consequence an accelerator action of the respiratory mechanism of reaction be required—in other words, a rapid series of thrusts and relaxations of the abdominal wall musculature instead of one strong steady thrust. These thrusts and relaxations would take place with the chest full of air, and the excess of air would not be emptied out until the effort was over—in other words, "rest breathing expiration" would not take place till reaction breathing had been abandoned altogether.

The Study of Breathlessness in the Patient.—The first thing that strikes the observer in watching a breathless patient is the fact that he seems incapable of holding his breath. The patient himself says that he is "short of wind," and amplifies the statement by the remark that he "hasn't enough

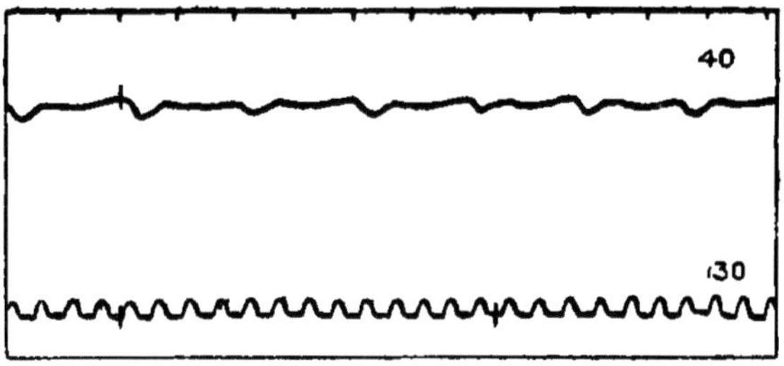

FIG. 38.—Note twitch of recti muscles at each inspiration.

breath for the effort." He is nevertheless respiring rapidly and his chest is expanded and full of air all the time, both in inspiration and expiration—these acts being exceedingly "shallow" and not seeming to affect the bulk of air in his chest. Only when the effort ends or is abandoned does he "let the air out" of his chest and "stop to breathe" himself. Moreover, the shape of the chest during the breathlessness occurring with effort is noteworthy. The chest is pulled open, *the abdomen is drawn in.* In other words, the picture of Reaction Breathing is present. In

Fig. 38 (which came from a boy in apparent collapse and was so taken that the tambour of the respiratory tracing apparatus was placed on abdomen) it is seen how the recti muscles twitched at the end of each inspiration—the respiratory rate was 40 and there was very little respiratory wave (pulse also showed pure acceleration and was 130). This is an illustration of respiratory acceleration. So also are the cases of so-called "paroxysmal dyspnœa," of which Fig. 39 furnishes an illustration (respiration rate, 80).

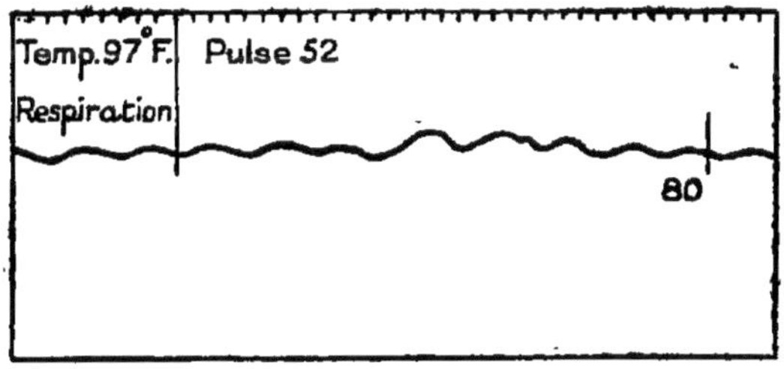

FIG. 39.—Paroxysmal Dyspnœa. Respiration Rate, 80. Pulse Rate, 52.

Dyspnœa will occur in Bed when the Vagus Depressor Mechanism becomes hyperexcitable.—It is evident from the foregoing that breathlessness is a phenomenon of respiration comparable to acceleration in the circulatory system and appearing when special efforts are required to overcome special emergencies. So that if the vagus depressor should from any cause become so extremely excitable that the ordinary plane of living in bed could no longer be maintained without effort, breathlessness in bed would and does result. The patient, in order to maintain his ordinary plane and compensate for his vagus depressor hyperexcitability, would first augment and then accelerate his breathing, as shown in the diagram (Fig. 40), where the arrows mark the beginning of vagus depressor pull, and its accentuation. (Figs. 41, 42, 43, and 44 also illustrate this point.) The writer saw one case in which a respiratory rate of 180 fell to 20 under hypnotism. He was able to make a tracing of the case, but unfortunately parted with it. The fall was abrupt, as the patient, who was

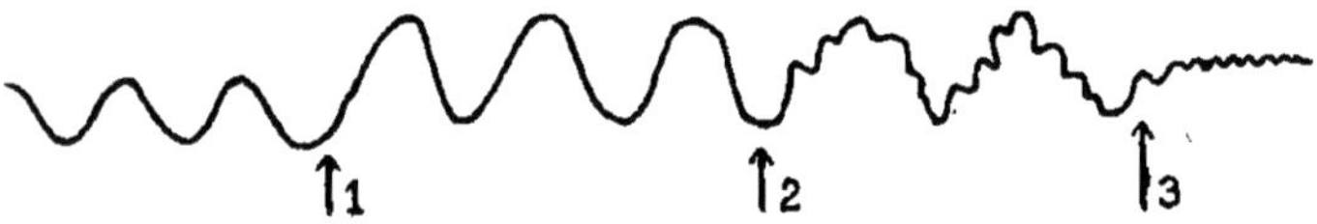

FIG. 40.—Augmentation and Acceleration of Respiration.

intensely frightened, yielded to suggestion. The quick rate began as sharply as ever the instant the man was awakened. The effect of hypnotism was evidently to prevent the stimuli of life from acting on a hyperexcitable vagus depressor mechanism. The moment the stimuli began to exert their force again the symptoms returned unabated.

Breathlessness is a Nervous Phenomenon.— Lewis and Cotton suggested a chemical basis for the breathlessness of D.A.H.—to wit, a lowering of "buffer salt" content in the blood. This work was based upon the findings of Barcroft. While nothing is further from the writers' intention than to contest the results obtained by these

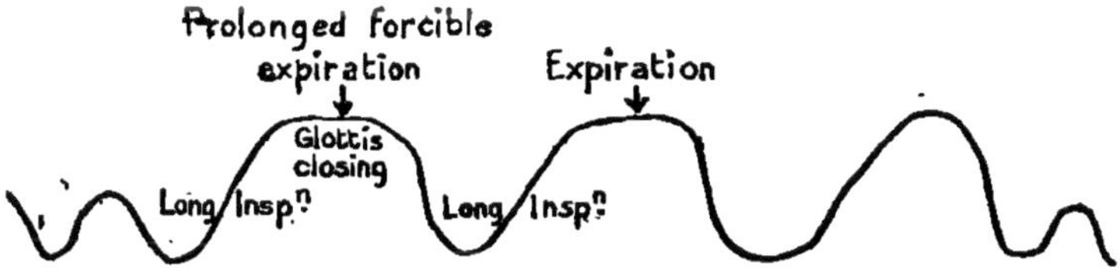

FIG. 41.—This and succeeding figures show in what manner, during increasing vagal hyper-irritability, augmented breathing gives place to accelerated breathing, the one rhythm being superimposed on the other.

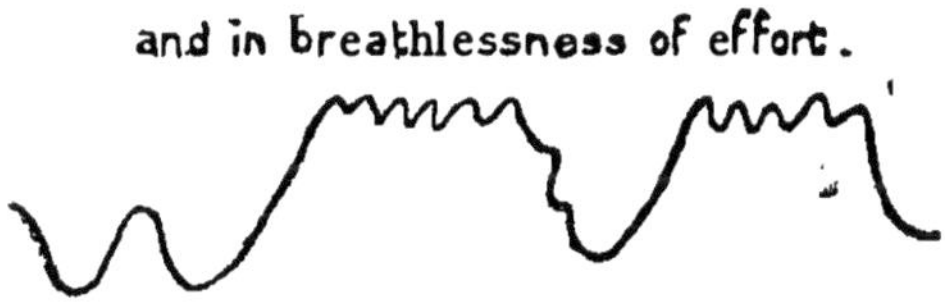

FIG. 42.

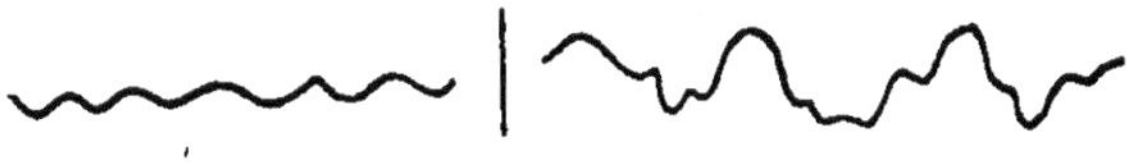

FIG. 43.

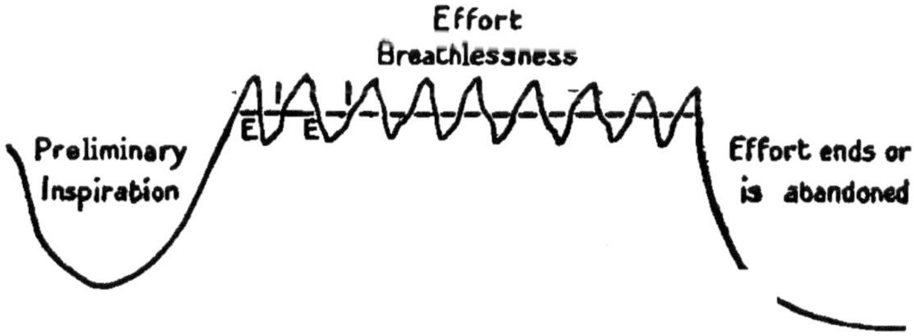

FIG. 44.

extremely brilliant and successful investigators, it is necessary to point out that they did not exclude from their paper the possibility that a lowered " buffer salt " content may be a result rather than a cause of the symptom sought to be explained in terms of it.

On the other hand, as we have seen, a hyper-excitable state of the vagus depressor mechanism is a sufficient explanation of the phenomena observed, and affords a clear idea why those phenomena arise, how they arise, and in what circumstances they arise. The extreme rapidity of the onset of breathlessness after a stimulus, *e.g.* after a fright, seems to cast additional doubt upon any purely chemical explanation. The breathlessness indeed, like the tachycardia, is a compensatory phenomenon. The patient is struggling to achieve an effect. The moment that effect is achieved breathlessness disappears.

CHAPTER IX

GIDDINESS

UP till now we have spoken of a pressor effect as a necessity of effort or rather of reaction. We must therefore further study this effect and define what we mean by it. In the first place, it must be made clear that a mechanism exists in the body whereby, in answer to a call for effort, whether physical or mental, blood is transferred in greater amount to the brain or muscles, or both. This mechanism normally consists of, first, a gradual closing of the blood lakes or hearts —what we have called "plus-systole"; secondly, of an augmented beating of the lakes or hearts; and, finally, of an acceleration of their rate of beating —three distinct mechanisms having a most beautiful interdependence and all tending to the same end. Indeed the production of plus-systole or closure of the lakes is a part of augmentation, for it occurs as the abscissa or each succeeding diastole rises under the influence of increasing sympathetic response.

If the vagus depressor is normal, acceleration will, as we have seen, be of moderate extent at all times that it is present. If, on the contrary, the vagus depressor is slightly hyperexcitable more acceleration will occur. If it is very excitable acceleration will have to be dropped and slowing will occur. Further excitability will upset the mechanism of augmentation and once more acceleration will occur, until a point is reached beyond which even acceleration will fail to support life.

Manifestly even slight hyperexcitability of the vagus will mean therefore a restricted field of effort—and also excessive response to small calls for effort. The victim will react maximally to minimal stimuli, maximal stimuli will find him unable to react at all, because not even his most extreme degree of acceleration will provide an adequate response to the overwhelming vagus depressor pull. If he is very "ill" he may be unable to leave his bed, because the mere effort of standing is for him an effort above his powers of reaction. Yet in bed he will be developing maximal reactions to the smallest trifles of his imagination or surroundings, and so be excited and to all appearances active and restless. If the process goes still further, even excitement in bed may be beyond the reach of his powers of reaction.

Now it has been found that pressure in arteries rises during the periods of blood transference, *i.e.* during effort or excitement. Consequently, in patients who are able to undertake a given effort, *i.e.* to make an adequate response by augmentation, or augmentation and acceleration, variations in pulse rate during the effort should not affect blood pressure to any great extent. The desired result is achieved—at one moment by slow, powerful beats, at another by quicker beats. The blood has been transferred and is being kept where it is required. The pressure remains more or less even. (For example, if a very small dose of atropine, *e.g.* $\frac{1}{200}$ grain be given and the pulse thereby slowed in a case of functional heart disease—that is to say, if the need for acceleration be lessened—the systolic blood pressure reading will not alter. In a case of the writer's the pulse rate was 90 before $\frac{1}{200}$ grain, atropine subcutaneously. In twenty minutes after the dose the pulse was 65. The blood pressure at 90 pulse rate was 140 systolic and 90 diastolic; at 65 pulse rate the blood pressure was also 140 systolic and 90 diastolic.)

When maximal reaction follows minimal stimuli—for example, the small stimuli of everyday life—then rapid pulse rate and relatively high blood pressures will be encountered apparently without much cause (*e.g.* 140 to 170 systolic with pulse rates of 90 to 140 and even higher); when maximal stimuli are applied to these cases and the vagus depressor is thus more powerfully affected, response will fail and a lower instead of higher blood pressure than obtained before the stimulus was applied may be encountered, and the effort will not succeed—on the contrary, what are usually spoken of as "symptoms of collapse" will show themselves.

A high pressure, then, with tachycardia when the effort in hand is an insignificant one indicates that maximal responses are being made to minimal stimuli; and that indicates that maximal stimuli will in all probability evoke insufficient responses.

Blood Pressure Responses to Maximal Stimuli in Functional Heart Disease.—These insufficient responses may be accompanied by—

1. A decided fall of pressure.
2. A rise of pressure less than the maximal rise when the stimulus is minimal.
3. No change of pressure.

A decided fall will occur when the stimulus so acts upon the hyperexcited vagus depressor as to occasion a violent "pull," and thus to prevent for the moment, or permanently, a reciprocal compensating pull of the sympathetic. The patient may faint away or may merely feel giddy.

A rise of pressure will occur when the vagus depressor pull is less violent (either because the vagus depressor mechanism is less excited or because the stimulus is less severe). The sympathetic compensation will be present but will be inadequate, and the raised pressure will only indicate a half-performed function. The patient will feel giddy and weak.

No change of pressure clearly falls between these other two.

Giddiness, then, is an expression of insufficient response to meet a particular demand. Like tachycardia, breathlessness, and palpitation it will therefore occur at one time and not at another, its occurrence at any given time being determined by the state of excitement of the vagus depressor mechanism and the strength of the stimulus.

Giddiness occurs with a Rise of Pressure as well as a Fall.—Once this is grasped it is seen how incomplete is the explanation of giddiness which ascribes it to a sudden "fall of intracerebral pressure"—*e.g.* on assuming the standing posture. Giddiness, as Lewis points out, may occur with a rise of pressure. We add that *when it does, that rise will be found to be less than the rise of pressure seen in the same patient in response to the same stimulus at times when he is able to react to it easily*—i.e. *without experiencing any unpleasant sensation.*

Lewis writes :—

"But the question of postural giddiness in these soldiers is not always so simple as might appear from this account. There are instances of giddiness in which an excessive fall of blood pressure on standing is not to be observed; moreover, there are rarer instances where giddiness is also experienced on lying down. . . . Where soldiers have complained of spontaneous giddiness while standing, the blood pressure during the period of giddiness has sometimes been found reduced, but in several instances it has been raised (by as much as 20 or 25 mm.)."

Giddiness on lying down is comparable to Giddiness at

the End of Effort.—Giddiness is often complained of at the end of effort—that is to say, when the sympathetic response weakens and the blood is transferred back to its lakes. The vagus depressor if it is excitable comes back sharply and with greater force than normal—on the principle that action and reaction are equal and opposite. The blood may be so sharply drawn back from brain and muscles that the amount required for the minor activities of rest may not be left in these organs—giddiness (or even fainting and collapse) will at once occur. In the same way, when a man lies down he virtually reduces his response and the vagus depressor is in consequence released from sympathetic reaction for the moment. If it is too active, and so by opening the blood lakes too suddenly withdraws too much blood from the brain, giddiness will follow no matter what the blood pressure may be like at the moment (the blood pressure in the arms, of course, will show a rise owing to removal of gravity). In other words, whatever reading the blood pressure instrument may show, is too low a reading for the immediate necessity of the case if giddiness occurs.

The Law of Giddiness.—Giddiness occurs, then, whenever cerebral blood pressure is inadequate to the needs of the moment. It occurs with pressures at, above, and below the resting normal. *But when it occurs with a raised pressure that pressure is less than the pressure at which the patient can* *perform the same action or mental process without discomfort.*

We may conclude this chapter with another quotation from Lewis :—

"If patient and control undertake an amount of work which in each produces the same degree of respiratory distress (the patient therefore doing less work), then the blood pressure reached and the amount of the rise is the same in the average for patient and control."

CHAPTER X

PRÆCORDIAL PAIN

IT will be observed that patients who suffer from præcordial pain usually complain that this symptom occurs during effort or just after effort—in other words, at or about the times that giddiness is complained of. The pain is felt over the præcordial area and varies from a dull ache to a sharp anginous stab which may pass down the left arm. The pain is frequently accompanied by an area of hyperalgesia of the skin over the left breast.

Meakins and Gunson, working at Mount Vernon, showed that the hyperalgesic areas vary from time to time in the same patient, and further that they increase with a rise of temperature and get smaller when the febrile manifestation is over.

Lewis, discussing the pain, writes :—

"In almost all patients who complain of uneasiness or actual pain it is provoked or intensified by exercise of any kind; pain rarely occurs at rest."

Hyperalgesia or tenderness was noted by Meakins and Gunson to be especially frequent in patients with a history of rheumatic fever or a recent history of other infectious disease. They found also that—" *The capacity for work of cases which present hyperalgesia is low.*"

Pain occurs at the Moment when Sympathetic Response to Vagus Depressor Pull fails to achieve the Necessary Effect.— From the foregoing it will be evident that the location of this *moment* in time and circumstances is very variable. We may give a few examples:—

1. A patient with functional heart disease is asked to bring a bucket of coals, and does so easily; pulse being 120 per minute and blood pressure 140.

   He is then told that his afternoon leave has been stopped and is instructed to fetch another bucket of coals. He now experiences pain and giddiness. Pulse 130; B.P. 130.

   Here the additional vagus depressor stimulation is supplied by the depressing news from outside that his leave has been stopped. In consequence the vagus depressor is more irritable and responds more vigorously. The sympathetic is unable to overcome this, even by acceleration to 130. The B.P. falls 10 mm. Hg, and pain and giddiness with palpitation and some dyspnœa come on.

2. A patient with temperature 98°·4 is invited to perform a stair test—ascending twenty steps—and does so without difficulty. His temperature rises to 99°·8 and then the symptoms, giddiness, pain, palpitation, and dyspnœa come on.

   Here the additional vagus stimulation is supplied by his own toxin.

3. A patient is asked to carry a weight and does so easily. He is then asked to carry double the weight and has symptoms as above.

   Here the additional vagus stimulation is supplied by the greater effort (stimulus to effort).

4. A patient is unable to ascend stairs without symptoms: he is given a *small* dose of atropine and thereafter performs the act without trouble.

   The vagus depressor excitability has been reduced by atropine (and the pulse has fallen from 90 to 74 on account of that reduction).

Pain, then, is an Expression of Failure.—This follows. But it cannot be too firmly insisted on that failure may occur in the same man at the same task one day and not another, one hour and not another, one instant and not another. Unless all the factors governing the situation are considered, this will seem inexplicable. The chief factors are (and these are but a few of them) :—

1. The state of vagus excitability.

   This is affected by—

   a. Toxins (*e.g.* trench fever toxins from bowel, etc.).

   b. Weather (*e.g.* damp weather increases the excitability possibly by increasing the susceptibility of sensory organs to stimulation and so exaggerating stimuli.

   c. Surroundings, " atmosphere," companions, emotions, mental states (*e.g.* fear of returning to battle front).

   d. Food and drink.

2. The nature of stimuli received.

   To some extent this is a part of 1.*c.* above—that is to say, that any call for effort following the receipt of bad news (itself a call for effort or stimulus) will find a more irritable vagus than it would have found had it come before the receipt of the bad news. In cases where the first stimulus (*e.g.* receipt of bad news; shell explosion) has been of very great severity and has acted upon a vagus depressor already rendered hyperexcitable by a toxin, the resulting vagus excitability may have been so great that the patient may have " fainted "—*i.e.* failed to react at all. *In that case no further stimuli will produce any reaction at all for the time.*

These factors, then, determine the reactions or failure of reactions of the patient to the manifold activities and stimuli of life. In addition there is the factor of habit, mental and physical, habitual activities always being easier than unaccustomed ones. But failure of complete reaction, no matter how produced or in what circumstances, is attended by dyspnœa, giddiness, palpitation, and præcordial pain.

The Relief of Præcordial Pain signifies the Completion of Reaction or its Abandonment.—It is easy to observe how patients who suffer pain on beginning an effort frequently get rid of the pain if they continue the effort. Their response is delayed, in other words, but is not impossible of realization, given time and perseverance.

The abandonment of effort or reaction is different a little, because reaction cannot quite be abandoned so long as stimuli remain. Forgetfulness and " memory block " are the means employed by many sufferers, but if the attention of these is called to the vetoed subject, præcordial pain, giddiness, flushing, and other signs may come on forthwith. These people may be said to have "fainted along a particular nerve path." They resent being awakened along that path and suffer acutely if they are.

The Nature of Præcordial Pain.—If careful investigations are made it will be found that præcordial pain never occurs as an isolated symptom; when it is present there are always other symptoms present, *e.g.* tightness of the chest and dyspnœa, abdominal disturbances and pain, giddiness, weakness, and so forth. These symptoms are local expressions of "want," and there seems to be no difficulty in accepting the præcordial pain and hyperalgesia—which is often widespread—as a local expression also (*i.e.* as an expression of cardiac "want") of the inability of the heart to perform the needful work.

This, however, is not at all necessarily a myocardial matter. In functional heart disease it is certainly never a myocardial matter. It is a nervous matter: the sympathetic is overwhelmed by the vagus depressor; systolic activity is insufficient to overcome diastolic so as to "deliver the goods" in the amount required by the demand of the moment.

Mackenzie has suggested that hyperalgesia over the præcordium is a phenomenon depending on segmental overexcitability, and so is an expression on the skin of the cardiac distress (see diagram, Fig. 45). Thus the local insufficiency in the heart is reflected on the local skin area. But hyperalgesia areas are by no means confined to the skin of the præcordium. In toxic cases they may extend over the whole body covering, that is to say, the whole muscular field. We then speak of "myalgia."

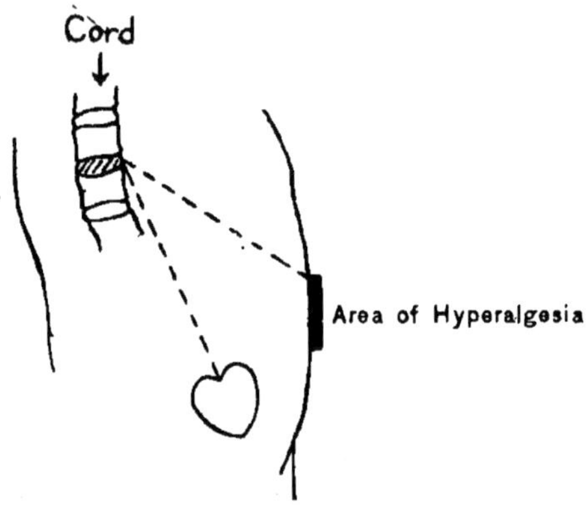

FIG. 45.—Illustrating Mackenzie's View of the Mechanism of Hyperalgesia of the Skin over the Præcordium.

They are very variable, like all the symptoms of this condition, but they follow the general rule: the greater the distress (the greater the failure) the greater is the extent of hyperalgesia.

CHAPTER XII

FLUSHING, BLUSHING, AND VASOMOTOR PHENOMENA

ALL the victims of functional heart disease show in a greater or less degree what are usually called "vasomotor disturbances." They blush and pale easily, they exhibit white lines on stroking the skin (white tache), or bright red lines with white borders (red tache), and in cold weather they often have blue or even black hands. Sometimes when stripped they seem to be cyanosed all over the skin, at other times what is called "chain-mail" cyanosis is observed.

These are phenomena of the skin or peripheral blood lake. We have already discussed the general behaviour of this lake at great length. It remains to point out that the lake is so constructed that any small part of it may respond to stimuli, without other parts which are not stimulated being affected. This truth was indicated by the writer in *The Hearts of Man*, and can be seen diagrammatically in the Fig. 46.

The stimulus affects only five of the skin hearts

(arterioles, capillaries, etc.), and these then go into plus-diastole.

1. If this is moderate in extent a local augmentation occurs, and the part *gets red* with quickly moving blood.
2. If this is more extreme in extent a local stasis occurs, and the part gets blue, because augmentation is insufficient to make up for the diastolic pull. The blood moves slowly.

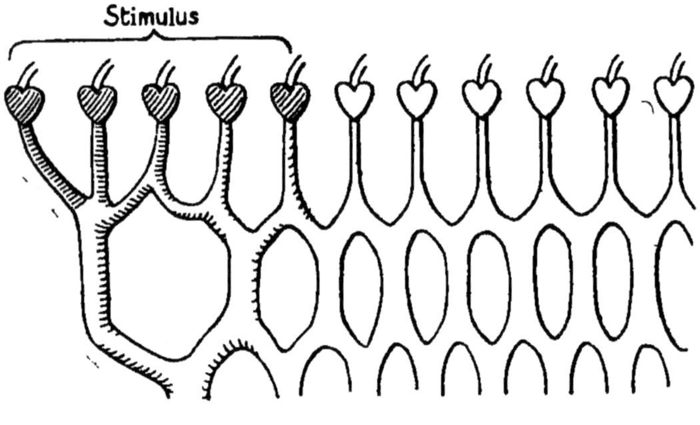

FIG. 46.—Illustrating the Localization of Stimuli to small Peripheral Vascular Areas.

In *The Hearts of Man* it was suggested that during diastolic states peristalsis in the arteries connecting the hearts (the so-called systemic arteries) is more active. Occasionally when the local area is in wide diastole, local arterial peristalsis becomes so great to this area that the arteries *are shut* (Fig. 47), then the area will go dead white, and the Raynaud's picture be produced. In Raynaud's disease we are presented with the picture of a red, a white, and a blue finger quite frequently. Raynaud's conditions are common in functional heart disease.

The reason why these phenomena are most frequently seen in the hands is because the hands are exposed to stimuli from which the other parts

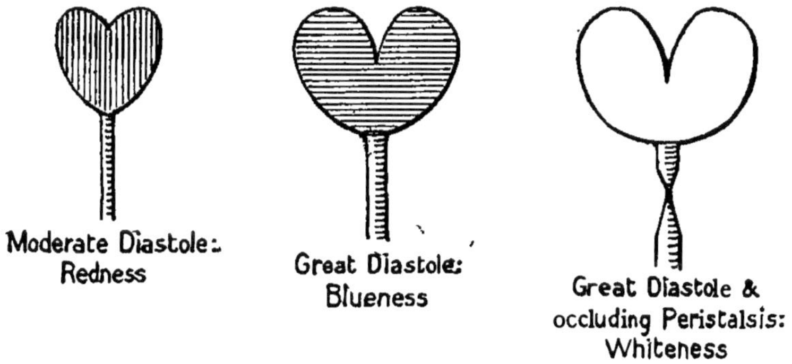

FIG. 47.—The Three Pictures of Raynaud's Disease.

of the body are protected. If the body be stripped, the phenomena will be seen to occur wherever stimuli occur. Thus, slapping the skin of the body lightly with a cold cloth will induce a cyanotic colour in the area slapped in cases where the hands are blue.

CHAPTER XII

Pulse Rate and Fever in Functional Heart Disease

IT will be found that the rate of the heart by no means always affords an indication of temperature in cases of functional heart disease. For example, a patient with a quick pulse may have a temperature of 99° F.; a patient with a pulse of 80 may have a temperature of 101°·5 F., and so on. This disparity must be considered with some care, because, as we have suggested, the excitability of the vagus depressor mechanism seems to determine both the pulse rate and the temperature, and it is consequently difficult to understand why pulse and temperature do not habitually move together.

The difficulty becomes less if we realize what in fact a temperature in these cases means: it means that a condition of *excessive diastole* with a consequent stasis of blood in the radiators has occurred and has not been fully compensated or responded to by the sympathetic. Full compensation by the sympathetic will reduce the temperature to normal, *other things being equal.*

When the pulse in these cases of temperature (101°·5) runs about 90 we must therefore conclude that the systolic or sympathetic response is below the requirements of the situation (*i.e.* the hyper-excitable vagus). We shall find on taking the blood pressure that it will tend in these cases to be a little below the usual normal (*e.g.* normal 130 B.P. now 110). If the toxin goes on outpouring, the temperature will rise and the pulse perhaps move a little slower; the blood pressure will continue to fall. In other words, with the temperature at 101 and the pulse at 90 and the B.P. at 110, the sympathetic effort being made was maximal —a further vagus pull strains this sympathetic effort still further, and now acceleration will tend to occur. Excessive rapidity (130) with a small tension pulse represents thus a sympathetic response of a maximal but inadequate character. The pressure falls further and the patient is in grave danger.

But a turn for the better now may occur. The toxin no longer outflows and the temperature falls, the pulse may slow down at once to a very low rate, comparatively speaking, though the blood pressure which is now creeping up has not yet reached normal. There is no longer so strong a vagus pull as to prevent augmentation—in other words, the *excessive diastole* has become less excessive and so the response has become more adequate. The temperature falls.

If, on the other hand, the toxin still slightly outflows, the pulse will remain accelerated even after the temperature has come down. In short, if the vagus release is complete at the "crisis," pulse and temperature will become normal and stay normal. If it is not complete, the crisis will not be a complete crisis and the pulse will remain accelerated to compensate for the vagus pull which remains. On this being released the pulse will fall to normal. If toxin outflows slightly, the pulse rate will again accelerate.

The accompanying chart-diagram attempts to show this (Fig. 48). It must be understood, however, that the slowing shown before the sharp rise in pulse rate is not always present in life, the acceleration often tending, on the contrary, to enter the picture at once. The determining factor is the rate of the outflow of toxin and the virulence of the toxin.

The Quick Pulse of Fever and the Quick Pulse of Effort are functionally Different though fundamentally the same.—Before showing some charts we may emphasize that this quick pulse of fever differs from the quick pulse of effort in the respect that *the acceleration in fever is a means of struggling up to normal; the acceleration in effort is a means of rising above normal.*

In effort vagus pull is *over compensated* and the blood pressure rises; in fever and toxic states of the vagus depressor generally the vagus pull is not over but *under compensated* to a greater or less

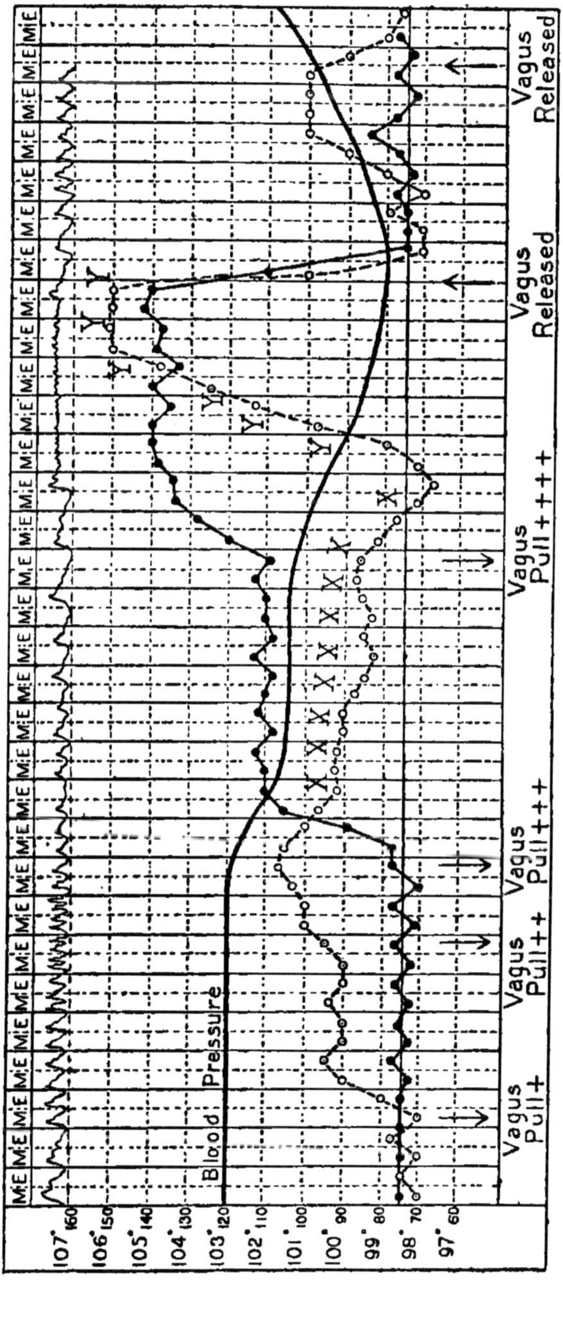

FIG. 48.—Chart-Diagram to illustrate Relation of Pulse Rate to Temperature and Blood Pressure in Fever.

extent and the blood pressure either remains normal (complete compensation) or falls (incomplete compensation).

In the chart-diagram (Fig. 48) this is graphically shown. It will be seen that at the first outpouring of toxin (Vagus Pull +) the pulse accelerates and the pressure remains unaffected. The temperature does not rise. A further outpouring (Vagus ++ and Vagus +++) quickens the pulse still further; but this response is now insufficient, and the temperature rises and the B.P. falls. The pulse now slows somewhat, the vagus pull being stronger than the measure of response, *i.e.* acceleration is rendered difficult. Next, a still greater outflow occurs (Vagus Pull ++++) and we have a sharp fall of pressure. The pulse shoots away up. It might be thought that as slowing had succeeded acceleration in the first instance on the toxin outflow becoming greater this new acceleration must differ in quality from the first form of acceleration. This, however, is not the case. In the first acceleration, an adequate response, we had both augmentation and increased rapidity. A further raising of vagus hyperexcitability slows the pulse by raising the load imposed on the sympathetic response. This can no longer maintain its augmentation and acceleration and the latter is dropped. On these terms a fairly good response can still be kept up. But a further outpouring of toxin still further raises hyperexcitability of the vagus depressor. This entirely unhinges the reciprocal arrangement between vagus and sympathetic which makes up the mechanism of augmentation. Now only by an intense acceleration can life be maintained.

There is thus a point in vagus hyperexcitability at which quickening will occur, a further point at which slowing will succeed to quickening, and a still further point at which great quickening will succeed to slowing, with a sharp fall of B.P. Figs. 49, 50, and 51 illustrate this by showing the varying effects of deep inspiration on the pulse at various temperatures. In Figs. 50 and 51 the vagus was very irritable, and the blood pressure fell markedly when the breath was taken.

In studying the effects of atropine, this complicated mechanism of response must be borne in mind. If it is not understood, atropine becomes a drug the action of which is well-nigh inexplicable; if it is understood, atropine is recognized as a drug of most definite and certain effect in reducing the excitability of the vagus depressor—in other words, in neutralizing the effects of the toxins producing functional heart disease. Though, as will appear later, its brief action renders it not very suitable for treatment.

A Study of Functional Heart Disease Charts.—In Fig. 52 from a case with trench fever (outset of attack) the above points are illustrated. In this chart the toxin at first slows the pulse,

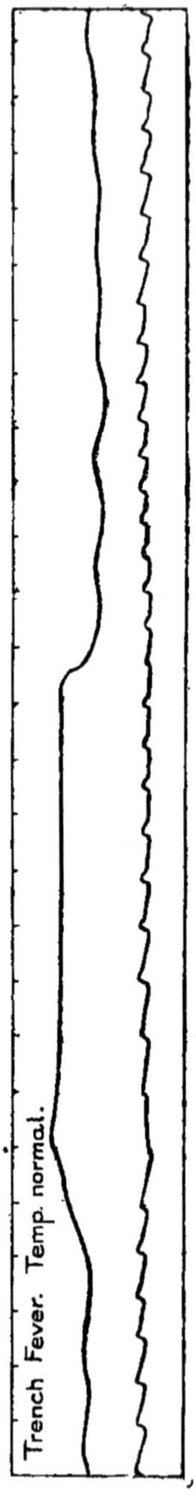

FIG. 49.—Small Effect of Deep Inspiration. Temperature Normal.

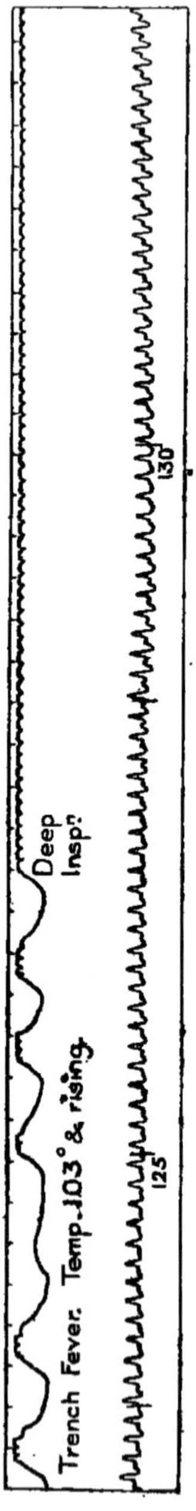

FIG. 50.—There was a Marked Fall of Blood Pressure on Deep Inspiration.—The rate did not vary much, as it was already very fast and the pulse of low tension.

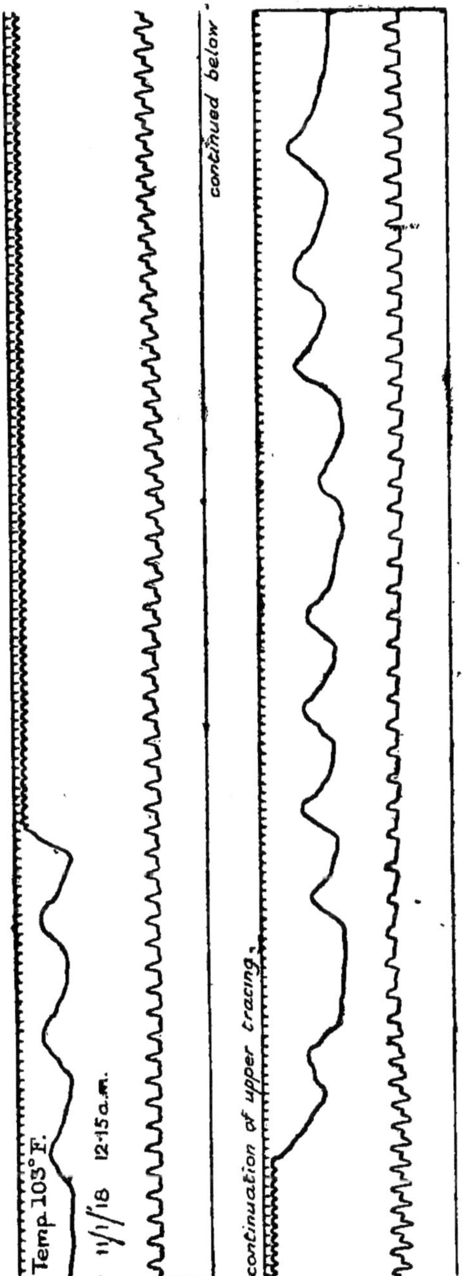

FIG. 51.—Marked Fall of Blood Pressure on Deep Inspiration.

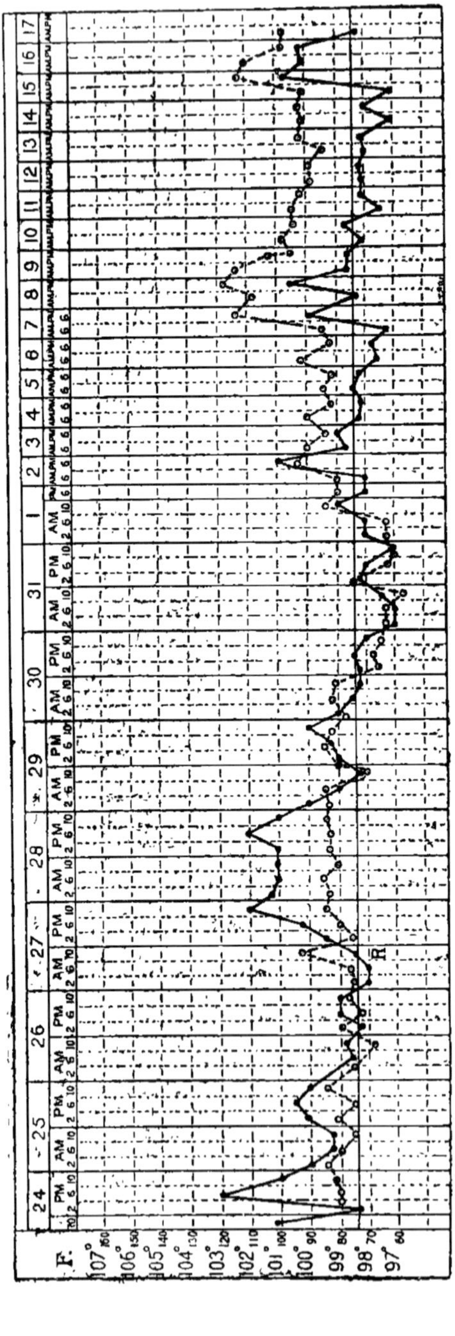

FIG. 52.—Temperature and Pulse in Trench Fever.

response being poor at the beginning in this individual case. The temperature falls (*i.e.* the toxin stops) and then another outpouring begins. This time the response is much more vigorous and speedy and the pulse runs off (point R) in order to compensate the vagus pull, but the compensation is not nearly enough and so the temperature rises and the pulse is held down (B.P. rather low, 110). However, on the next attack the mechanism of compensation has become better established, and the pulse rate rises steadily

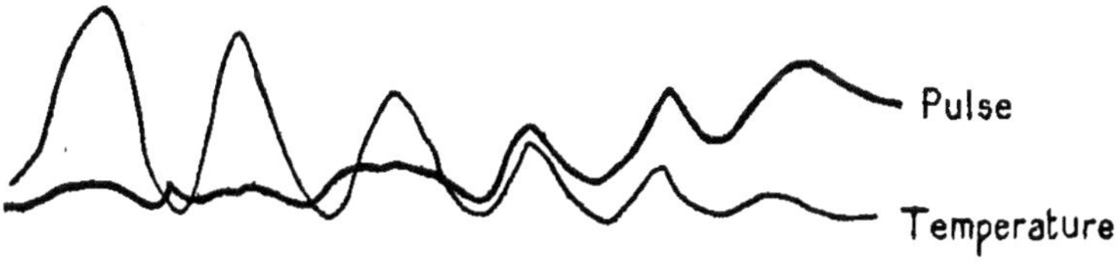

FIG. 53.—As Pulse Rate rises, Temperature tends to stabilize.

when vagus pull begins, *so that a rapid pulse is obtained with a relatively low temperature and a relatively high pressure* (Fig. 53). In other words, the temperature shows a declining height across the chart, the pulse an ascending height; stasis is thus prevented and cooling facilitated. (See chapter on "Temperature.") Compensation is being increased and established.

When the temperature and pulse reach their new relationship—*i.e.* when compensation is established—active life can once more be lived, *though on a lowered plane.* This is also seen in Fig. 54.

In some cases no early slowing is noted, an active

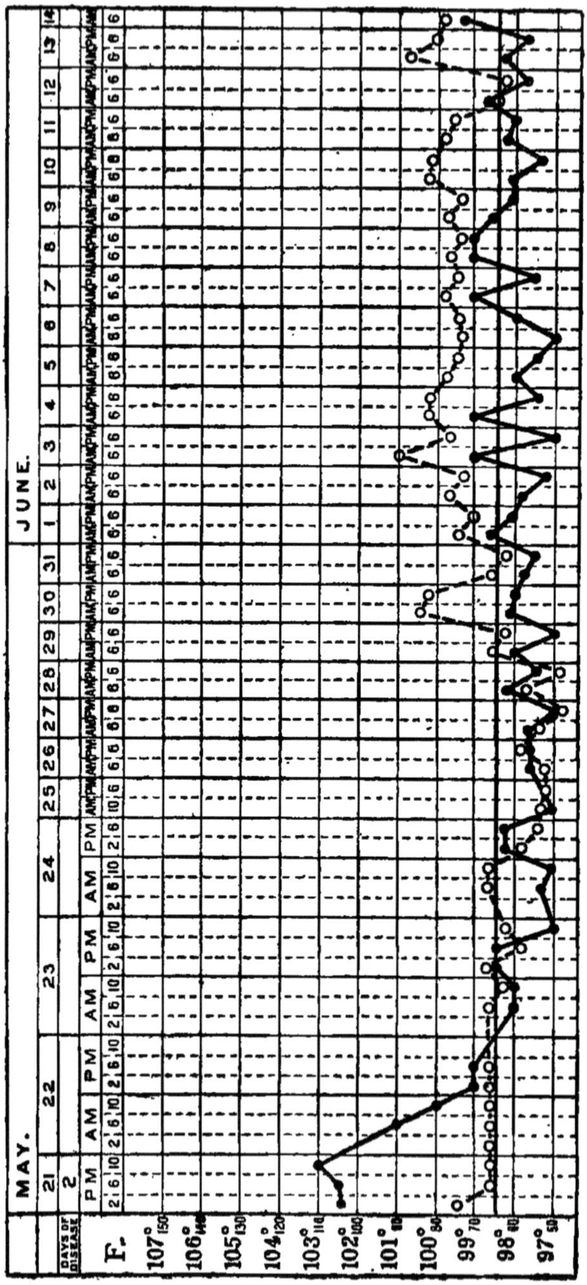

FIG. 54.—Showing the Gradual Domination of Pulse over Temperature.

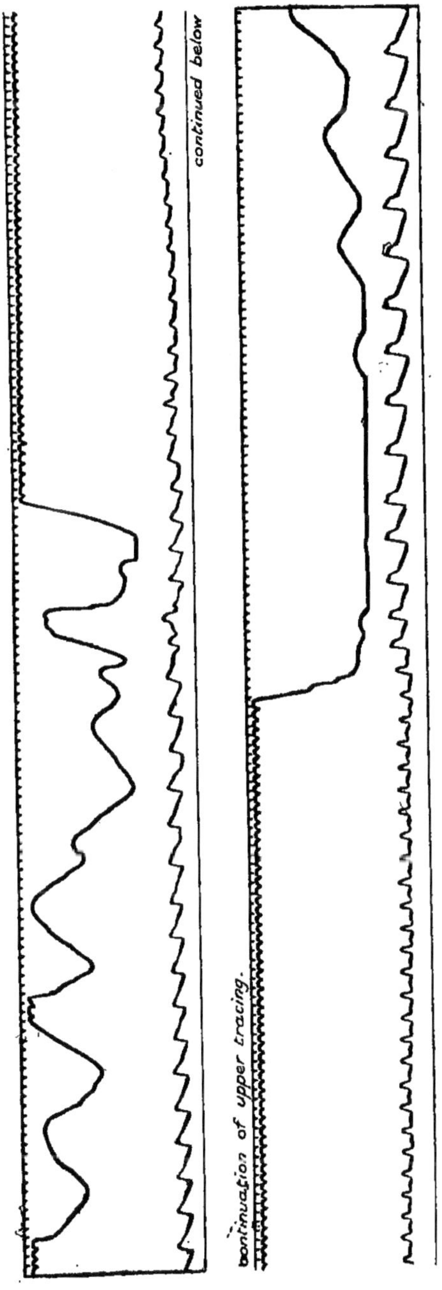

FIG. 55.—Sharp Fall of Blood Pressure in case of Trench Fever with Hyperexcitable Vagus on Deep Inspiration.

response with acceleration occurring. These may run an afebrile course. In this chart the acceleration is always of the first type described above. But if during the slow-pulse period a deep inspiration was taken and the vagus thus strongly stimulated, the intense rapidity of the second type of acceleration occurred at once (*vide* Fig. 55) with a sharp fall of B.P.

CHAPTER XIII

PROGNOSIS

THE prognosis in functional heart disease will depend evidently upon the nature of the cause of that disease. As we have seen, any of the circumstances of life may cause the symptoms if these circumstances produce an excitable enough condition of the vagus depressor mechanism. But in actual practice it will be found that men and women who are not subject to any toxæmia do not display the symptoms to a marked degree, or for any considerable length of time, even in circumstances of the most severe strain. Consequently it is probable that the vast majority of cases of functional heart disease are toxic in origin. The nature of the toxin will therefore determine the prognosis in most instances.

After diseases like pneumonia, symptoms similar to those of functional heart disease manifest themselves; but as convalescence passes on, and the patient regains his strength, the symptoms go away. The attack has been "recovered from," the pneumococcus no longer exercises its effects,

The same applies to a great number of other illnesses, *e.g.* septic conditions, diphtheria, etc., after which the patients tend to be dyspnœic on exertion, have palpitation, are giddy, and suffer from præcordial pain. In all these instances the prognosis is good and the symptoms of functional heart disease may be expected to disappear, provided the patient is a healthy individual.

When "Rheumatism" or Trench Fever is the Cause of Functional Heart Disease the Prognosis so far as Cure is concerned is Bad.—Very different is the picture in those cases which are called "rheumatic" or those in which trench fever is definitely the cause of the condition. In these it seems very probable that the infection persists—as indeed was suggested by Mackenzie and as some recent work under Major Byam on trench fever has shown (lice fed on a case of "neurasthenia" following trench fever at an interval of two years were able to transmit the original disease). The question of prognosis therefore is really a question of the extent of the compensation effected between hyperexcitable vagus depressor and sympathetic.

The stethoscope will afford very little assistance here, though it is a fact that many of the patients present an apical systolic murmur, and that the left border of the heart is frequently found in the nipple line or just outside it. A more reliable test is the response to an effort test—for example, climbing twenty steps. The following points should be noted :—

1. Breathlessness.
2. Palpitation.
3. Giddiness.
4. Præcordial pain.
5. Pulse rate.

When the first four are markedly present and the pulse rate is greatly increased and remains high for a considerable period, *e.g.* more than 3 or 4 minutes, the outlook is unfavourable in the absence of treatment.

The fallacies of this test are, however, numerous. For example, the patient may have a raised temperature, in which case he will at the moment be toxic beyond his everyday normal. The temperature should therefore always be taken before the test is made, and if it is 99° F. or above that, the test should be postponed.

Again, the patient may be greatly worried and excited at the moment, and this will tend to exaggerate his response. Consequently, the confidence of the patient must be secured, and his circumstances understood so far as possible before the test is carried out.

The weather, too, exercises a pronounced effect, a falling barometer constituting a snare : the test will always give an exaggerated result when the barometer is falling or low. Gastric disturbances and alcohol also may affect the readings obtained.

A further test from which useful information is to be obtained is that carried out by means of a long deep inspiration. The patient is instructed to take a long deep breath and hold it as long as he can. The pulse is felt. It will be found that *in afebrile cases* of moderate severity the pulse will slow somewhat, *e.g.* 10 to 20 beats per minute; in more severe cases the slowing will be greater, and in still more severe cases an initial slowing of a few beats will give way suddenly to marked *loss of volume and acceleration.* Still more severity will show no slowing, but only loss of volume and acceleration. Finally, complete disappearance of the pulse at the wrist may be encountered. When the test is carried out the patient should be seated and should have been seated for some time—ten minutes at least.

If the temperature is raised or rising, no test should be performed. Indeed, the fallacies which apply to the effort test apply to this one. A falling temperature is also apt to be misleading, so that a clear day of afebrile state should intervene after a temperature spike before any test is applied.

When the response to effort is bad and the pulse test gives a sharp fall of volume in afebrile periods the outlook in untreated cases is not good. These patients are practically "decompensated" in a nervous sense. Their field of effort is very greatly restricted. But until treatment has been tried thoroughly no prognosis should be made, and it should further always be borne in mind that, as frequently happens, the toxin may enter on a period of " latency " at any time and the patient become surprisingly much better in consequence. Nevertheless, if the cases be followed, a measure of restriction of effort will be found to persist in the vast majority of them, and " relapses " are almost inevitable.

CHAPTER XIV

PRINCIPLES OF TREATMENT

THE treatment of functional heart disease clearly falls into two categories :—

1. The treatment of the infection causing the disease.
2. Palliative treatment.

The treatment of infections cannot be dealt with in such a volume as this. But the case cited by Sir James Mackenzie, in which removal of a diseased appendix cured the heart condition of the patient, illustrates the lines of action suggested. In cases of functional heart disease following scarlet fever, diphtheria, and other acute conditions, cure may be expected if and when the infection dies out. Cases following amœbic dysentery have, as has been stated, been cured by bismuth-emetine-iodide. On the other hand, cases following or accompanying tuberculosis, rheumatic conditions, and trench fever have proved incurable in the real sense, because these infections have remained incurable in the majority of instances. Until the infections are brought within the range of curative treatment, palliation remains the physician's only method of dealing with them.

The Object of Palliative Treatment of Functional Heart Disease is Increase of Sympathetic Activity or of "Response."—It has emerged from our study that functional heart disease is no more than exhaustion—that is to say, than incapacity to meet the demands of life. The mechanism of the exhaustion depends on the fact that a toxin acting upon the vagus depressor system has rendered that system hyperexcitable, and so imposed upon the sympathetic system an additional strain. Small stimuli evoke full responses; to great calls for effort, response is either impossible or incomplete. It is manifest that measures which will—

a. Lower the irritability of the vagus depressor system, or

b. increase the resources of the sympathetic system,

will act as palliatives in these cases by increasing the activity of response.

Evidently the first duty of the physician will be to relieve his patient of " depressing " circumstances—that is to say, of external and also of mental factors tending to increase vagus depressor irritability. One of the chief of these factors will almost invariably be found to be fear of " heart disease." Victims of functional heart conditions are painfully aware of their symptoms and take a grave view of them. They are too frequently encouraged in this attitude by their medical advisers, who may have detected a systolic murmur or an extra-systole or other supposed danger sign. The patient learns that his heart is "weak" and at once begins to take an interest in this organ; he begins to rest himself, to avoid effort, to resent calls upon his activities. If his doctor supports him, he becomes an invalid forthwith.

The first thing to do with this man is to disabuse his mind of the idea that his heart is diseased, and as a general rule this can only be done by affording him a rational explanation of his symptoms. Mere assurances are useless, for in all probability he has other medical opinions to place against these optimistic views. He jumps to the conclusion that he is merely being "let down easily." The physician should be quite candid and quite explicit. The writers begin as a rule by calling the patient's attention to his generally flabby state—the flabby state of his muscles, of his abdominal muscles in particular. They mention casually that the heart also is a muscle and must be expected to share in the general flabbiness. They then explain how the blood supply of the muscles and brain is conditioned by the abdominal musculature as well as by the heart itself, and suggest that the giddy sensations which bulk so large in the patient's fears are due to accumulation of blood in the abdomen at the expense of the brain. The idea of heart disease is thus merged in the idea of general lack of tone, and thus it is comparatively easy to indicate the toxic nature of the condition —" the system is poisoned," the heart merely suffers along with other members. If the patient is interested in motors he may be told that it is not the engine which is at fault, but the spark, the timing. " The nerves to the muscles and heart are poisoned." (The use of the term nervousness or neurasthenia should be avoided, as this at once arouses antagonism.)

So soon as the patient grasps the idea that he is the victim of a poisoned nervous system and that herein lies the cause of his sensations, he will ask if tonics cannot be given him, and the names of much-advertised proprietary preparations will rise to his mind. He must be told that not all but only certain of his nerves are affected, and that indiscriminate taking of tonics may be harmful. His position is like that of a " machine running with the brakes on." The problem to be solved in his case is how to take the brakes off.

He will then be in a fit state of mind to realize that fear of his own condition is one of the worst enemies he has to fight, and this realization will go far to dispel his fear and so to restore his mind to equilibrium and to its normal activity.

The immediate result will be a question as to how much effort may be undertaken with safety.

9

The answer should at once be given, "As much as you care to make." There is no danger in effort: the danger lies in rest. An arm kept in a sling wastes; and the same applies to a heart. Hearts, like other muscles, become more useful by exercise and training. And thus also perhaps may the poison be worked out of the "system."

The patient will now adopt a new view of life and of his condition, and thus a huge burden will be removed from his shoulders. Graduated exercises of one kind or another may now be ordered, or, better still, the playing of games enjoined, or the enjoyment of sports like fishing or shooting recommended. This as a preliminary to return to work. The object should be declared to be "to develop and strengthen the flabby muscles and so counteract and dispel the poison." A further object, which need not be insisted upon, because the less the patient thinks about it the better, is to occupy the mind and prevent brooding.

Finally, a tonic treatment may properly be prescribed, it being insisted upon that this is no "heart medicine" in the narrow sense.

The Best Tonic in Functional Heart Disease is Thyroid Extract. — The work of Levy has proved that thyroid increases the pressor effects of adrenalin 300 to 400 per cent. This drug in the writers' hands has given remarkable results, and Captain Carroll, who was the first to recommend its use in these cases, has had especially good results with it. The best dose is 1 grain daily to begin with, but this may be increased to 8 or even 10 grains daily in accordance with the needs of the individual case. Marked slowing has been the rule in cases of tachycardia.

Atropine may also be used, but the results are not so good as when thyroid is employed. The patients, as might be expected, show a remarkable tolerance to the drug, and as much as $\frac{1}{33}$ grain thrice daily by mouth fails in most instances to dilate the pupil even after ten days of continuous administration. In a few cases a combination of atropine, $\frac{1}{100}$ grain thrice daily, and thyroid, 1 grain daily, has proved a satisfactory method of handling the cases.

No other drugs have been of service, and digitalis is notably useless in these cases. Under thyroid, however, and with a mind set at rest, the patient often makes what appears to be a complete recovery, more especially if he is freed from anxieties.

If the patient is wealthy, a dry climate may be recommended; and if an outdoor life is possible, it is a help towards recovery. But the writers are opposed to the policy of altering a man's career on account of this condition. The city worker can get all the exercise he requires in the vast majority of cases. To uproot him and transplant him to the country is a mistake. The mental upheaval occasioned is likely to be attended by so much distress and anxiety that any good obtained is discounted in advance. Moreover, the stimulus of an accustomed mode of life is valuable; friendships are valuable; ambitions are valuable. Drastic change of occupation usually means a loss of all three.

The writers do not forbid their patients to smoke, nor yet to take alcohol. They believe that the irritation caused by these prohibitions is much more harmful than the pleasures themselves. They do not diet their patients, though the advice given by Sir James Mackenzie in some cases—to abstain from butter and fats—has proved very helpful in their experience. Once again, interference with established habit appears to them to be fraught with danger. The less the patient is encouraged to think of himself as an invalid the more rapid and complete is his recovery likely to be.

INDEX

Spotted something that isn't quite right?

Let us know and we'll fix it for future reprints. And as a thank you for your diligence, we'll send you a free Sothis book of your choice.

publisher@sothis.press

This page intentionally left blank